Practice the HESI A2!

Health Information Systems
Practice Test Questions

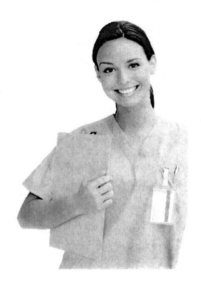

Test Preparation Publishing
Victoria BC Canada

the production of, and does not endorse, this product.

ISBN-13: 978-1-928077-57-2

Version 6.5 February 2015

Published by
Complete Test Preparation Inc.
921 Foul Bay Rd.
Victoria BC Canada V8S 4H9
Visit us on the web at http://www.test-preparation.ca
Printed in the USA

About Complete Test Preparation

The Complete Test Preparation Team has been publishing high quality study materials since 2005. Thousands of students visit our websites every year, and thousands of students, teachers and parents all over the world have purchased our teaching materials, curriculum, study guides and practice tests.

Complete Test Preparation is committed to provide students with the best study materials and practice tests available on the market. Members of our team combine years of teaching experience, with experienced writers and editors, all with advanced degrees.

Team Members for this publication

Editor: Brian Stocker MA
Contributor: Dr. C. Gregory
Contributor: Dr. G. A. Stocker DDS
Contributor: D. A. Stocker M. Ed.
Contributor: Dr. N. Wyatt

Feedback

We welcome your feedback. Email us at feedback@test-preparation.ca with your comments and suggestions. We carefully review all suggestions and often incorporate reader suggestions into upcoming versions. As a Print on Demand Publisher, we update our products frequently.

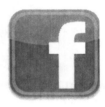 **Find us on Facebook**

www.facebook.com/CompleteTestPreparation

Contents

Getting Started

CONGRATULATIONS! By deciding to take the Health Education Systems (HESI® A2) Exam, you have taken the first step toward a great future! Of course, there is no point in taking this important examination unless you intend to do your very best in order to earn the highest grade you possibly can. That means getting yourself organized and discovering the best approaches, methods and strategies to master the material. Yes, that will require real effort and dedication on your part but if you are willing to focus your energy and devote the study time necessary, before you know it you will be opening that letter of acceptance to the school of your dreams.

We know that taking on a new endeavour can be a little scary, and it is easy to feel unsure of where to begin. That's where we come in. This study guide is designed to help you improve your test-taking skills, show you a few tricks of the trade and increase both your competency and confidence.

The Health Education Systems A2® Exam

The HESI® A2 exam is composed of modules and not all schools use all of the modules. It is therefore very important that you find out what modules your school will use! That way you won't waste valuable study time learning something that isn't on your exam!

The HESI® A2 Modules are: Mathematics, Vocabulary, Reading Comprehension, English grammar, and a Science module which includes, Biology, Chemistry, Physics, Basic Scientific principals and Anatomy and Physiology.

You don`t have to worry because these sections are included in this study guide. However, to maximize your study time, it is very important to check which modules your university offers before studying everything under the sun!

While we seek to make our guide as comprehensive as possible, note that like all entrance exams, the HESI® A2 Exam might be adjusted at some future point. New material might be added, or content that is no longer relevant or applicable might be removed. It is always a good idea to give the materials you receive when you register to take the HESI® a careful review.

The HESI® Study Plan

Now that you have made the decision to take the HESI, it's time to get started. Before you do another thing, you will need to figure out a plan of attack. The very best study tip is to start early! The longer the time period you devote to regular study practice, the more likely you will retain the material and be able to reach it quickly. If you thought that 1x20 is the same as 2x10, guess what? It really is not, when it comes to study time. Reviewing material for just an hour per day over the course of 20 days is far better than studying for two hours a day for only 10 days. The more often you revisit a particular piece of information, the better you will know it. Not only will your grasp and understanding be better, but your ability to reach into your brain and quickly and efficiently pull out the tidbit you need, will be greatly enhanced as well.

The great Chinese scholar and philosopher Confucius believed that true knowledge could be defined as knowing what you know and what you do not know. The first step in preparing for the HESI® Exam is to assess your strengths and weaknesses. You may already have an idea of what you know and what you do not know, but evaluating yourself using our Self-Assessment modules for each of the three areas, math, english science and reading, will clarify the details.

Making a Study Schedule

To make your study time most productive, you will need to

develop a study plan. The purpose of the plan is to organize all the bits of pieces of information in such a way that you will not feel overwhelmed. Rome was not built in a day, and learning everything you will need to know to pass the HESI® Exam is going to take time, too. Arranging the material you need to learn into manageable chunks is the best way to go. Each study session should make you feel as though you have accomplished your goal, and your goal is simply to learn what you planned to learn during that particular session. Try to organize the content in such a way that each study session builds on previous ones. That way, you will retain the information, be better able to reach it, and review the previous bits and pieces at the same time.

Self-assessment

The Best Study Tip! The very best study tip is to start early! The longer you study regularly, the more you will retain and 'learn' the material. Studying for 1 hour per day for 20 days is far better than studying for 2 hours for 10 days.

What don't you know?

The first step is to assess your strengths and weaknesses. You may already have an idea of where your weaknesses are, or you can take our Self-assessment modules for each of the areas, math, English, science and reading.

Below is a table to assess your exam readiness in each content area. You can fill this in now, and correct if necessary after completing the self-assessments, or fill it in after you have taken the self-assessments.

Self-assessment

The Best Study Tip! The very best study tip is to start early! The longer you study regularly, the more you will retain and 'learn' the material. Studying for 1 hour per day for 20 days is far better than studying for 2 hours for 10 days.

What don't you know?

The first step is to assess your strengths and weaknesses. You may already have an idea of where your weaknesses are, or you can take our Self-assessment modules for each of the areas, Math, English, Science and Reading Comprehension.

Exam Component	Rate 1 to 5
Reading Comprehension	
Paragraph & Passage Comprehension	
Drawing inferences & conclusions	
English Grammar	
Vocabulary	
Math	
Fractions	
Decimals	
Percent	
Word Problems	
Basic Algebra	
Science	
Anatomy and Physiology	
Biology	
Chemistry	

Making a Study Schedule

The key to making a study plan is to divide the material you need to learn into manageable size and learn it, while at the same time reviewing the material that you already know.

Using the table above, any scores of 3 or below, you need to spend time learning, going over and practicing this subject area. A score of 4 means you need to review the material, but you don't have to spend time re-learning. A score of 5 and you are OK with just an occasional review before the exam.

A score of 0 or 1 means you really need to work on this area and should allocate the most time and the highest priority. Some students prefer a 5-day plan and others a 10-day plan. It also depends on how much time you have until the exam.

Here is an example of a 5-day plan based on an example from the table above:

Fractions: 1 Study 1 hour everyday – review on last day
Biology: 3 Study 1 hour for 2 days then ½ hour a day, then review
Vocabulary: 4 Review every second day
Word Problems: 2 Study 1 hour on the first day – then ½ hour everyday
Reading Comprehension: 5 Review for ½ hour every other day
Algebra: 5 Review for ½ hour every other day
Chemistry: 5 very confident – review a few times.

Using this example, Chemistry and Grammar are good and only need occasional review. Biology is also good and needs 'some' review. Decimals need a bit of work, Word Problems need a lot of work and Fractions are very weak and need the majority of time. Based on this, here is a sample study plan:

Day	Subject	Time
Monday		
Study	Fractions	1 hour
Study	Word Problems	1 hour
	½ hour break	
Study	Biology	1 hour
Review	Chemistry	½ hour
Tuesday		
Study	Fractions	1 hour
Study	Word Problems	½ hour
	½ hour break	
Study	Decimals	½ hour
Review	Vocabulary	½ hour
Review	Grammar	½ hour
Wednesday		
Study	Fractions	1 hour
Study	Word Problems	½ hour
	½ hour break	
Study	Biology	½ hour
Review	Chemistry	½ hour
Thursday		
Study	Fractions	½ hour
Study	Word Problems	½ hour
Review	Biology	½ hour
	½ hour break	
Review	Grammar	½ hour
Review	Vocabulary	½ hour

Friday		
Review	Fractions	½ hour
Review	Word Problems	½ hour
Review	Biology	½ hour
	½ hour break	
Review	Vocabulary	½ hour
Review	Grammar	½ hour

Practice Test Questions Set 1

Section I – Reading Comprehension

Questions: 45
Time: 60 Minutes

Section II – Mathematics

Questions: 50
Time: 60 Minutes

Section III English Grammar

Questions: 50
Time: 50 Minutes

Section IV - Vocabulary

Questions: 50
Time: 50 Minutes

Section V – Part I – Science

Questions: 75
Time: 125 minutes

Section VI Anatomy & Physiology

Questions: 25
Time: 25 minutes

The questions below are not the same as you will find on the HESI® - that would be too easy! And nobody knows what the questions will be and they change all the time. Below are general questions that cover the same subject areas as the HESI. While the format and exact wording of the questions may differ slightly, and change from year to year, if you can answer the questions below, you will have no problem with the HESI.

For the best results, take this Practice Test as if it were the real exam. Set aside time when you will not be disturbed, and a location that is quiet and free of distractions. Read the instructions carefully, read each question carefully, and answer to the best of your ability.

Use the bubble answer sheets provided. When you have completed the Practice Test, check your answer against the Answer Key and read the explanation provided.

Do not attempt more than one set of practice test questions in one day. After completing the first practice test, wait two or three days before attempting the second set of questions.

This set of practice test questions contains ALL of the HESI® modules. Different schools use different modules so be sure to check with your school for the modules being used.

Reading Comprehension

1. (A) (B) (C) (D)

2. (A) (B) (C) (D)

3. (A) (B) (C) (D)

4. (A) (B) (C) (D)

5. (A) (B) (C) (D)

6. (A) (B) (C) (D)

7. (A) (B) (C) (D)

8. (A) (B) (C) (D)

9. (A) (B) (C) (D)

10. (A) (B) (C) (D)

11. (A) (B) (C) (D)

12. (A) (B) (C) (D)

13. (A) (B) (C) (D)

14. (A) (B) (C) (D)

15. (A) (B) (C) (D)

16. (A) (B) (C) (D)

17. (A) (B) (C) (D)

18. (A) (B) (C) (D)

19. (A) (B) (C) (D)

20. (A) (B) (C) (D)

21. (A) (B) (C) (D)

22. (A) (B) (C) (D)

23. (A) (B) (C) (D)

24. (A) (B) (C) (D)

25. (A) (B) (C) (D)

26. (A) (B) (C) (D)

27. (A) (B) (C) (D)

28. (A) (B) (C) (D)

29. (A) (B) (C) (D)

30. (A) (B) (C) (D)

31. (A) (B) (C) (D)

32. (A) (B) (C) (D)

33. (A) (B) (C) (D)

34. (A) (B) (C) (D)

35. (A) (B) (C) (D)

36. (A) (B) (C) (D)

37. (A) (B) (C) (D)

38. (A) (B) (C) (D)

39. (A) (B) (C) (D)

40. (A) (B) (C) (D)

41. (A) (B) (C) (D)

42. (A) (B) (C) (D)

43. (A) (B) (C) (D)

44. (A) (B) (C) (D)

45. (A) (B) (C) (D)

Mathematics

1. (A) (B) (C) (D)   18. (A) (B) (C) (D)   35. (A) (B) (C) (D)

2. (A) (B) (C) (D)   19. (A) (B) (C) (D)   36. (A) (B) (C) (D)

3. (A) (B) (C) (D)   20. (A) (B) (C) (D)   37. (A) (B) (C) (D)

4. (A) (B) (C) (D)   21. (A) (B) (C) (D)   38. (A) (B) (C) (D)

5. (A) (B) (C) (D)   22. (A) (B) (C) (D)   39. (A) (B) (C) (D)

6. (A) (B) (C) (D)   23. (A) (B) (C) (D)   40. (A) (B) (C) (D)

7. (A) (B) (C) (D)   24. (A) (B) (C) (D)   41. (A) (B) (C) (D)

8. (A) (B) (C) (D)   25. (A) (B) (C) (D)   42. (A) (B) (C) (D)

9. (A) (B) (C) (D)   26. (A) (B) (C) (D)   43. (A) (B) (C) (D)

10. (A) (B) (C) (D)   27. (A) (B) (C) (D)   44. (A) (B) (C) (D)

11. (A) (B) (C) (D)   28. (A) (B) (C) (D)   45. (A) (B) (C) (D)

12. (A) (B) (C) (D)   29. (A) (B) (C) (D)   46. (A) (B) (C) (D)

13. (A) (B) (C) (D)   30. (A) (B) (C) (D)   47. (A) (B) (C) (D)

14. (A) (B) (C) (D)   31. (A) (B) (C) (D)   48. (A) (B) (C) (D)

15. (A) (B) (C) (D)   32. (A) (B) (C) (D)   49. (A) (B) (C) (D)

16. (A) (B) (C) (D)   33. (A) (B) (C) (D)   50. (A) (B) (C) (D)

17. (A) (B) (C) (D)   34. (A) (B) (C) (D)

English Grammar

1. (A) (B) (C) (D)
2. (A) (B) (C) (D)
3. (A) (B) (C) (D)
4. (A) (B) (C) (D)
5. (A) (B) (C) (D)
6. (A) (B) (C) (D)
7. (A) (B) (C) (D)
8. (A) (B) (C) (D)
9. (A) (B) (C) (D)
10. (A) (B) (C) (D)
11. (A) (B) (C) (D)
12. (A) (B) (C) (D)
13. (A) (B) (C) (D)
14. (A) (B) (C) (D)
15. (A) (B) (C) (D)
16. (A) (B) (C) (D)
17. (A) (B) (C) (D)

18. (A) (B) (C) (D)
19. (A) (B) (C) (D)
20. (A) (B) (C) (D)
21. (A) (B) (C) (D)
22. (A) (B) (C) (D)
23. (A) (B) (C) (D)
24. (A) (B) (C) (D)
25. (A) (B) (C) (D)
26. (A) (B) (C) (D)
27. (A) (B) (C) (D)
28. (A) (B) (C) (D)
29. (A) (B) (C) (D)
30. (A) (B) (C) (D)
31. (A) (B) (C) (D)
32. (A) (B) (C) (D)
33. (A) (B) (C) (D)
34. (A) (B) (C) (D)

35. (A) (B) (C) (D)
36. (A) (B) (C) (D)
37. (A) (B) (C) (D)
38. (A) (B) (C) (D)
39. (A) (B) (C) (D)
40. (A) (B) (C) (D)
41. (A) (B) (C) (D)
42. (A) (B) (C) (D)
43. (A) (B) (C) (D)
44. (A) (B) (C) (D)
45. (A) (B) (C) (D)
46. (A) (B) (C) (D)
47. (A) (B) (C) (D)
48. (A) (B) (C) (D)
49. (A) (B) (C) (D)
50. (A) (B) (C) (D)

Vocabulary

1. (A) (B) (C) (D)
2. (A) (B) (C) (D)
3. (A) (B) (C) (D)
4. (A) (B) (C) (D)
5. (A) (B) (C) (D)
6. (A) (B) (C) (D)
7. (A) (B) (C) (D)
8. (A) (B) (C) (D)
9. (A) (B) (C) (D)
10. (A) (B) (C) (D)
11. (A) (B) (C) (D)
12. (A) (B) (C) (D)
13. (A) (B) (C) (D)
14. (A) (B) (C) (D)
15. (A) (B) (C) (D)
16. (A) (B) (C) (D)
17. (A) (B) (C) (D)

18. (A) (B) (C) (D)
19. (A) (B) (C) (D)
20. (A) (B) (C) (D)
21. (A) (B) (C) (D)
22. (A) (B) (C) (D)
23. (A) (B) (C) (D)
24. (A) (B) (C) (D)
25. (A) (B) (C) (D)
26. (A) (B) (C) (D)
27. (A) (B) (C) (D)
28. (A) (B) (C) (D)
29. (A) (B) (C) (D)
30. (A) (B) (C) (D)
31. (A) (B) (C) (D)
32. (A) (B) (C) (D)
33. (A) (B) (C) (D)
34. (A) (B) (C) (D)

35. (A) (B) (C) (D)
36. (A) (B) (C) (D)
37. (A) (B) (C) (D)
38. (A) (B) (C) (D)
39. (A) (B) (C) (D)
40. (A) (B) (C) (D)
41. (A) (B) (C) (D)
42. (A) (B) (C) (D)
43. (A) (B) (C) (D)
44. (A) (B) (C) (D)
45. (A) (B) (C) (D)
46. (A) (B) (C) (D)
47. (A) (B) (C) (D)
48. (A) (B) (C) (D)
49. (A) (B) (C) (D)
50. (A) (B) (C) (D)

Science

1. (A) (B) (C) (D)   21. (A) (B) (C) (D)   41. (A) (B) (C) (D)   61. (A) (B) (C) (D)

2. (A) (B) (C) (D)   22. (A) (B) (C) (D)   42. (A) (B) (C) (D)   62. (A) (B) (C) (D)

3. (A) (B) (C) (D)   23. (A) (B) (C) (D)   43. (A) (B) (C) (D)   63. (A) (B) (C) (D)

4. (A) (B) (C) (D)   24. (A) (B) (C) (D)   44. (A) (B) (C) (D)   64. (A) (B) (C) (D)

5. (A) (B) (C) (D)   25. (A) (B) (C) (D)   45. (A) (B) (C) (D)   65. (A) (B) (C) (D)

6. (A) (B) (C) (D)   26. (A) (B) (C) (D)   46. (A) (B) (C) (D)   66. (A) (B) (C) (D)

7. (A) (B) (C) (D)   27. (A) (B) (C) (D)   47. (A) (B) (C) (D)   67. (A) (B) (C) (D)

8. (A) (B) (C) (D)   28. (A) (B) (C) (D)   48. (A) (B) (C) (D)   68. (A) (B) (C) (D)

9. (A) (B) (C) (D)   29. (A) (B) (C) (D)   49. (A) (B) (C) (D)   69. (A) (B) (C) (D)

10. (A) (B) (C) (D)   30. (A) (B) (C) (D)   50. (A) (B) (C) (D)   70. (A) (B) (C) (D)

11. (A) (B) (C) (D)   31. (A) (B) (C) (D)   51. (A) (B) (C) (D)   71. (A) (B) (C) (D)

12. (A) (B) (C) (D)   32. (A) (B) (C) (D)   52. (A) (B) (C) (D)   72. (A) (B) (C) (D)

13. (A) (B) (C) (D)   33. (A) (B) (C) (D)   53. (A) (B) (C) (D)   73. (A) (B) (C) (D)

14. (A) (B) (C) (D)   34. (A) (B) (C) (D)   54. (A) (B) (C) (D)   74. (A) (B) (C) (D)

15. (A) (B) (C) (D)   35. (A) (B) (C) (D)   55. (A) (B) (C) (D)   75. (A) (B) (C) (D)

16. (A) (B) (C) (D)   36. (A) (B) (C) (D)   56. (A) (B) (C) (D)

17. (A) (B) (C) (D)   37. (A) (B) (C) (D)   57. (A) (B) (C) (D)

18. (A) (B) (C) (D)   38. (A) (B) (C) (D)   58. (A) (B) (C) (D)

19. (A) (B) (C) (D)   39. (A) (B) (C) (D)   59. (A) (B) (C) (D)

20. (A) (B) (C) (D)   40. (A) (B) (C) (D)   60. (A) (B) (C) (D)

Anatomy and Physiology

1. Ⓐ Ⓑ Ⓒ Ⓓ   11. Ⓐ Ⓑ Ⓒ Ⓓ   21. Ⓐ Ⓑ Ⓒ Ⓓ

2. Ⓐ Ⓑ Ⓒ Ⓓ   12. Ⓐ Ⓑ Ⓒ Ⓓ   22. Ⓐ Ⓑ Ⓒ Ⓓ

3. Ⓐ Ⓑ Ⓒ Ⓓ   13. Ⓐ Ⓑ Ⓒ Ⓓ   23. Ⓐ Ⓑ Ⓒ Ⓓ

4. Ⓐ Ⓑ Ⓒ Ⓓ   14. Ⓐ Ⓑ Ⓒ Ⓓ   24. Ⓐ Ⓑ Ⓒ Ⓓ

5. Ⓐ Ⓑ Ⓒ Ⓓ   15. Ⓐ Ⓑ Ⓒ Ⓓ   25. Ⓐ Ⓑ Ⓒ Ⓓ

6. Ⓐ Ⓑ Ⓒ Ⓓ   16. Ⓐ Ⓑ Ⓒ Ⓓ

7. Ⓐ Ⓑ Ⓒ Ⓓ   17. Ⓐ Ⓑ Ⓒ Ⓓ

8. Ⓐ Ⓑ Ⓒ Ⓓ   18. Ⓐ Ⓑ Ⓒ Ⓓ

9. Ⓐ Ⓑ Ⓒ Ⓓ   19. Ⓐ Ⓑ Ⓒ Ⓓ

10. Ⓐ Ⓑ Ⓒ Ⓓ   20. Ⓐ Ⓑ Ⓒ Ⓓ

Section I - Reading Comprehension

Directions: The following questions are based on several reading passages. Each passage is followed by a series of questions. Read each passage carefully, and then answer the questions based on it. You may reread the passage as often as you wish. When you have finished answering the questions based on one passage, go right onto the next passage. Choose the best answer based on the information given and implied.

Questions 1 – 4 refer to the following passage.

Infectious Disease

An infectious disease is a clinically evident illness resulting from the presence of pathogenic agents, such as viruses, bacteria, fungi, protozoa, multi cellular parasites, and unusual proteins known as prions. Infectious pathologies are also called communicable diseases or transmissible diseases, due to their potential of transmission from one person or species to another by a replicating agent (as opposed to a toxin).

Transmission of an infectious disease can occur in many different ways. Physical contact, liquids, food, body fluids, contaminated objects, and airborne inhalation can all transmit infecting agents.

Transmissible diseases that occur through contact with an ill person, or objects touched by them, are especially infective, and are sometimes called contagious diseases. Communicable diseases that require a more specialized route of infection, such as through blood or needle transmission, or sexual transmission, are usually not regarded as contagious.

The term infectivity describes the ability of an organism to enter, survive and multiply in the host, while the infectiousness of a disease shows the comparative ease with which the disease is transmitted. An infection however, is not synonymous with an infectious disease, as an infection may not cause important clinical symptoms. [1]

1. What can we infer from the first paragraph in this passage?

a. Sickness from a toxin can be easily transmitted from one person to another.

b. Sickness from an infectious disease can be easily transmitted from one person to another.

c. Few sicknesses are transmitted from one person to another.

d. Infectious diseases are easily treated.

2. What are two other names for infections' pathologies?

a. Communicable diseases or transmissible diseases

b. Communicable diseases or terminal diseases

c. Transmissible diseases or preventable diseases

d. Communicative diseases or unstable diseases

3. What does infectivity describe?

a. The inability of an organism to multiply in the host.

b. The inability of an organism to reproduce.

c. The ability of an organism to enter, survive and multiply in the host.

d. The ability of an organism to reproduce in the host.

4. How do we know an infection is not synonymous with an infectious disease?

a. Because an infectious disease destroys infections with enough time.

b. Because an infection may not cause important clinical symptoms or impair host function.

c. We do not. The two are synonymous.

d. Because an infection is too fatal to be an infectious disease.

Questions 5 – 8 refer to the following passage.

Virus

A virus (from the Latin virus meaning toxin or poison) is a small infectious agent that can replicate only inside the living cells of other organisms. Most viruses are too small to be seen directly with a microscope. Viruses infect all types of organisms, from animals and plants to bacteria and single-celled organisms.

Unlike prions and viroids, viruses consist of two or three parts: all viruses have genes made from either DNA or RNA, all have a protein coat that protects these genes, and some have an envelope of fat that surrounds them when they are outside a cell. (Viroids do not have a protein coat and prions contain no RNA or DNA.) Viruses vary from simple to very complex structures. Most viruses are about one hundred times smaller than an average bacterium. The origins of viruses in the evolutionary history of life are unclear: some may have evolved from plasmids—pieces of DNA that can move between cells—while others may have evolved from bacteria.

Viruses spread in many ways; plant viruses are often transmitted from plant to plant by insects that feed on sap, such as aphids, while animal viruses can be carried by blood-sucking insects. These disease-bearing organisms are known as vectors. Influenza viruses are spread by coughing and sneezing. HIV is one of several viruses transmitted through sexual contact and by exposure to infected blood. Viruses can infect only a limited range of host cells called the "host range." This can be broad, as when a virus is capable of infecting many species or narrow. [2]

5. What can we infer from the first paragraph in this selection?

    a. A virus is the same as bacterium

    b. A person with excellent vision can see a virus with the naked eye

    c. A virus cannot be seen with the naked eye

    d. Not all viruses are dangerous

6. What types of organisms do viruses infect?

    a. Only plants and humans
    b. Only animals and humans
    c. Only disease-prone humans
    d. All types of organisms

7. How many parts do prions and viroids consist of?

    a. Two
    b. Three
    c. Either less than two or more than three
    d. Less than two

8. What is one common virus spread by coughing and sneezing?

    a. AIDS
    b. Influenza
    c. Herpes
    d. Tuberculosis

Questions 9 – 11 refer to the following passage.

Convection and Weather

The first stage of a thunderstorm is the cumulus stage, or developing stage. In this stage, masses of moisture are lifted upwards into the atmosphere. The trigger for this lift can be insulation heating the ground producing thermals, areas where two winds converge, forcing air upwards, or, where winds blow over terrain of increasing elevation. Moisture in the air rapidly cools into liquid drops of water, which appears as cumulus clouds.

As the water vapor condenses into liquid, latent heat is released which warms the air, causing it to become less dense than the surrounding dry air. The warm air rises in an updraft through the process of convection (hence the term convective precipitation). This creates a low-pressure zone beneath the forming thunderstorm. In a typical thunderstorm, approximately 5×10^8 kg of water vapor is lifted, and the quantity of energy released when this condenses is about equal to the energy used by a city of 100,000 in a month. [3]

9. The cumulus stage of a thunderstorm is the

   a. The last stage of the storm.

   b. The middle stage of the storm formation.

   c. The beginning of the thunderstorm.

   d. The period after the thunderstorm has ended.

10. One way the air is warmed is

   a. Air moving downwards, which creates a high-pressure zone.

   b. Air cooling and becoming less dense, causing it to rise.

   c. Moisture moving downward toward the earth.

   d. Heat created by water vapor condensing into liquid.

11. Identify the correct sequence of events.

   a. Warm air rises, water droplets condense, creating more heat, and the air rises further.

   b. Warm air rises and cools, water droplets condense, causing low pressure.

   c. Warm air rises and collects water vapor, the water vapor condenses as the air rises, which creates heat, and causes the air to rise further.

   d. None of the above.

Questions 12 – 14 refer to the following passage.

US Weather Service

The United States National Weather Service classifies thunderstorms as severe when they reach a predetermined level. Usually, this means the storm is strong enough to inflict wind or hail damage. In most of the United States, a storm is considered severe if winds reach over 50 knots (58 mph or 93 km/h), hail is ¾ inch (2 cm) diameter or larger, or if meteorologists report funnel clouds or tornadoes. In the Central Region of the United States National Weather Service, the hail threshold for a severe thunderstorm is 1 inch (2.5 cm) in diameter. Though a funnel cloud or tornado shows the presence of a severe thunderstorm, the various meteorological agencies would issue a tornado warning rather than a severe thunderstorm warning in this case.

Meteorologists in Canada define a severe thunderstorm as either having tornadoes, wind gusts of 90 km/h or greater, hail 2 centimeters in diameter or greater, rainfall more than 50 millimeters in 1 hour, or 75 millimeters in 3 hours.

Severe thunderstorms can develop from any type of thunderstorm. [3]

12. What is the purpose of this passage?

   a. Explaining when a thunderstorm turns into a tornado

   b. Explaining who issues storm warnings, and when these warnings should be issued

   c. Explaining when meteorologists consider a thunderstorm severe

   d. None of the above

13. It is possible to infer from this passage that

    a. Different areas and countries have different criteria for determining a severe storm.

    b. Thunderstorms can include lightning and tornadoes, as well as violent winds and large hail.

    c. If someone spots both a thunderstorm and a tornado, meteorological agencies will immediately issue a severe storm warning.

    d. Canada has a much different alert system for severe storms, with criteria that are far less.

14. What would the Central Region of the United States National Weather Service do if hail was 2.7 cm in diameter?

    a. Not issue a severe thunderstorm warning.

    b. Issue a tornado warning.

    c. Issue a severe thunderstorm warning.

    d. Sleet must also accompany the hail before the Weather Service will issue a storm warning.

Questions 15 – 18 refer to the following passage.

Clouds

A cloud is a visible mass of droplets or frozen crystals floating in the atmosphere above the surface of the Earth or other planetary bodies. Another type of cloud is a mass of material in space, attracted by gravity, called interstellar clouds and nebulae. The branch of meteorology which studies clouds is called nephrology. When we are speaking of Earth clouds, water vapor is usually the condensing substance, which forms small droplets or ice crystal. These crystals are typically 0.01 mm in diameter. Dense, deep clouds reflect most light, so they appear white, at least from the top. Cloud droplets scatter light very efficiently, so the farther into a cloud light travels, the weaker it gets. This accounts for the gray or dark appearance at the base of large clouds. Thin clouds may appear to have acquired the color of their environment or background. [4]

15. What are clouds made of?

    a. Water droplets

    b. Ice crystals

    c. Ice crystals and water droplets

    d. Clouds on Earth are made of ice crystals and water droplets

16. The main idea of this passage is

    a. Condensation occurs in clouds, having an intense effect on the weather on the surface of the earth.

    b. Atmospheric gases are responsible for the gray color of clouds just before a severe storm happens.

    c. A cloud is a visible mass of droplets or frozen crystals floating in the atmosphere above the surface of the Earth or other planetary body.

    d. Clouds reflect light in varying amounts and degrees, depending on the size and concentration of the water droplets.

17. The branch of meteorology that studies clouds is called

    a. Convection

    b. Thermal meteorology

    c. Nephology

    d. Nephelometry

18. Why are clouds white on top and grey on the bottom?

    a. Because water droplets inside the cloud do not reflect light, it appears white, and the further into the cloud the light travels, the less light is reflected making the bottom appear dark.

    b. Because water droplets outside the cloud reflect light, it appears dark, and the further into the cloud the light travels, the more light is reflected making the bottom appear white.

c. Because water droplets inside the cloud reflects light, making it appear white, and the further into the cloud the light travels, the more light is reflected making the bottom appear dark.

d. None of the above.

Questions 19 - 22 refer to the following recipe.

Low Blood Sugar

As the name suggest, low blood sugar is low sugar levels in the bloodstream. This can occur when you have not eaten properly and undertake strenuous activity, or, when you are very hungry. When Low blood sugar occurs regularly and is ongoing, it is a medical condition called hypoglycemia. This condition can occur in diabetics and also in healthy adults.

Causes of low blood sugar can include excessive alcohol consumption, metabolic problems, stomach surgery, pancreas, liver or kidneys problems, as well as a side-effect of some medications.

Symptoms

There are different symptoms depending on the severity of the case.

Mild hypoglycemia can lead to feelings of nausea and hunger. The patient may also feel nervous, jittery and have fast heart beats. Sweaty skin, clammy and cold skin are likely symptoms.

Moderate hypoglycemia can result in short temperedness, confusion, nervousness, fear and blurring of vision. The patient may feel weak and unsteady.

Severe cases of hypoglycemia can lead to seizures, coma, fainting spells, nightmares, headaches, excessive sweats and severe tiredness.

Diagnosis of low blood sugar

A doctor can diagnosis this medical condition by asking the patient questions and testing blood and urine samples. Home testing kits are available for patients to monitor blood sugar levels. It is important to see a qualified doctor though. The doctor can administer tests to ensure that will safely rule out other medical conditions that could affect blood sugar levels.

Treatment

Quick treatments include drinking or eating foods and drinks with high sugar contents. Good examples include soda, fruit juice, hard candy and raisins. Glucose energy tablets can also help. Doctors may also recommend medications and well as changes in diet and exercise routine to treat chronic low blood sugar.

19. Based on the article, which of the following is true?

    a. Low blood sugar can happen to anyone.

    b. Low blood sugar only happens to diabetics.

    c. Low blood sugar can occur even.

    d. None of the statements are true.

20. Which of the following are the author's opinion?

    a. Quick treatments include drinking or eating foods and drinks with high sugar contents.

    b. None of the statements are opinions.

    c. This condition can occur in diabetics and in healthy adults.

    d. There are different symptoms depending on the severity of the case

21. What is the author's purpose?

    a. To inform

    b. To persuade

    c. To entertain

    d. To analyze

22. Which of the following is not a detail?

a. A doctor can diagnosis this medical condition by asking the patient questions and testing.

b. A doctor will test blood and urine samples.

c. Glucose energy tablets can also help.

d. Home test kits monitor blood sugar levels.

Questions 23 – 25 refer to the following passage.

Keeping Tropical Fish

Keeping tropical fish as home or in your office used to be very popular. Today interest has declined, but it remains as rewarding and relaxing a hobby as ever. Ask any tropical fish hobbyist, and you will hear how soothing and relaxing watching colorful fish live their lives in the aquarium. If you are considering keeping tropical fish as pets, here is a list of the basic equipment that you will need.

A filter is essential for keeping your aquarium clean and your fish alive and healthy. There are different types and sizes of filters and the right size for you depends on the size of the aquarium and the level of stocking. Generally, you need a filter with a 3 to 5 times turn over rate per hour. This means that the water in the tank should go through the filter about 3 to 5 times per hour.

Most tropical fish do well in water temperatures ranging between 24C and 26C, though each has its own ideal water temperature. A heater with a thermostat is necessary to regulate the water temperature. Some heaters are submersible and others are not, so check carefully before you buy.

Lights are also necessary, and come in a large variety of types, strengths and sizes. A light source is necessary for plants in the tank to photosynthesize and give the tank a more attractive appearance. Even if you plan to use plastic plants, the fish still require light, although here you can use a lower strength light source.

A hood is necessary to keep dust, dirt and unwanted materials out of the tank. Sometimes the hood can also help prevent evaporation. Another requirement is aquarium gravel. This will help improve the aesthetics of the aquarium and is necessary if you plan to have real plants.

23. What is the general tone of this article?

    a. Formal

    b. Informal

    c. Technical

    d. Opinion

24. Which of the following can not be inferred?

    a. Gravel is good for aquarium plants.

    b. Fewer people have aquariums in their office than at home.

    c. The larger the tank, the larger the filter required.

    d. None of the above.

25. What evidence does the author provide to support their claim that aquarium lights are necessary?

    a. Plants require light.

    b. Fish and plants require light.

    c. The author does not provide evidence for this statement.

    d. Aquarium lights make the aquarium more attractive.

Questions 26 – 30 refer to the following passage.

Navy Seals

The United States Navy's Sea, Air and Land Teams, commonly known as Navy SEALs, are the U.S. Navy's principle special operations force, and a part of the Naval Special

Warfare Command (NSWC) as well as the maritime component of the United States Special Operations Command (USSOCOM).

The unit's acronym ("SEAL") comes from their capacity to operate at sea, in the air, and on land – but it is their ability to work underwater that separates SEALs from most other military units in the world. Navy SEALs are trained and have been deployed in a wide variety of missions, including direct action and special reconnaissance operations, unconventional warfare, foreign internal defence, hostage rescue, counter-terrorism and other missions. All SEALs are members of either the United States Navy or the United States Coast Guard.

In the early morning of May 2, 2011 local time, a team of 40 CIA-led Navy SEALs completed an operation to kill Osama bin Laden in Abbottabad, Pakistan about 35 miles (56 km) from Islamabad, the country's capital. The Navy SEALs were part of the Naval Special Warfare Development Group, previously called "Team 6." President Barack Obama later confirmed the death of bin Laden. The unprecedented media coverage raised the public profile of the SEAL community, particularly the counter-terrorism specialists commonly known as SEAL Team 6. [5]

26. Are Navy SEALs part of USSOCOM?

    a. Yes

    b. No

    c. Only for special operations

    d. No, they are part of the US Navy

27. What separates Navy SEALs from other military units?

    a. Belonging to NSWC

    b. Direct action and special reconnaissance operations

    c. Working underwater

    d. Working for other military units in the world

28. What other military organizations do SEALs belong to?

    a. The US Navy

    b. The Coast Guard

    c. The US Army

    d. The Navy and the Coast Guard

29. What other organization participated in the Bin Laden raid?

    a. The CIA

    b. The US Military

    c. Counter-terrorism specialists

    d. None of the above

30. What is the new name for Team 6?

    a. They were always called Team 6

    b. The counter-terrorism specialists

    c. The Naval Special Warfare Development Group

    d. None of the above

Questions 31 – 34 refer to the following passage.

Gardening

Gardening for food extends far into prehistory. Ornamental gardens were known in ancient times, a famous example being the Hanging Gardens of Babylon, while ancient Rome had dozens of gardens.

The earliest forms of gardens emerged from the people's need to grow herbs and vegetables. It was only later that rich individuals created gardens for purely decorative purposes.

In ancient Egypt, rich people created ornamental gardens to relax in the shade of the trees. Egyptians believed that gods liked gardens. Commonly, walls surrounded ancient Egyptian gardens with trees planted in rows.

The most popular tree species were date palms, sycamores, fig trees, nut trees, and willows. Besides ornamental gardens, wealthy Egyptians kept vineyards to produce wine.

The Assyrians are also known for their beautiful gardens in what we know today as Iraq. Assyrian gardens were very large, with some of them used for hunting and others as leisure gardens. Cypress and palm were the most popular trees in Assyrian gardens. [6]

31. Why did wealthy people in Egypt have gardens?

    a. For food

    b. To relax in the shade

    c. For ornamentation

    d. For hunting

32. What did the Egyptians believe about gardens?

    a. They believed gods loved gardens.

    b. They believed gods hated gardens.

    c. The didn't have any beliefs about gods and gardens.

    d. They believed gods hated trees.

33. What kinds of trees did the Assyrians like?

    a. The Assyrians liked date palms, sycamores, fig trees, nut trees, and willows.

    b. The Assyrians liked Cypresses and palms.

    c. The Assyrians didn't like trees.

    d. The Assyrians liked hedges and vines.

34. Which came first, gardening for vegetables or ornamental gardens?

> a. Ornamental gardens came before vegetable gardens.
>
> b. Vegetable gardens came before ornamental gardens.
>
> c. Vegetable and ornamental gardens appeared at the same time.
>
> d. The passage does not give enough information.

Questions 35 – 38 refer to the following passage.

The Civil War

The Civil War began on April 12, 1861. The first shots of the Civil War were fired in Fort Sumter, South Carolina. Note that even though more American lives were lost in the Civil War than in any other war, not one person died on that first day. The war began because eleven Southern states seceded from the Union and tried to start their own government, The Confederate States of America.

Why did the states secede? The issue of slavery was a primary cause of the Civil War. The eleven southern states relied heavily on their slaves to foster their farming and plantation lifestyles. The northern states, many of whom had already abolished slavery, did not think that the southern states should have slaves. The north wanted to free all the slaves and President Lincoln's goal was to both end slavery and preserve the Union. He had Congress declare war on the Confederacy on April 14, 1862. For four long, blood soaked years, the North and South fought.

From 1861 to mid 1863, it seemed as if the South would win this war. However, on July 1, 1863, an epic three day battle was waged on a field in Gettysburg, Pennsylvania. Gettysburg is remembered for being the bloodiest battle in American history. At the end of the three days, the North turned the tide of the war in their favor. The North then went onto dominate the South for the remainder of the war. Most well remembered might be General Sherman's "March to The Sea," where he famously led the Union Army through Georgia and the Carolinas, burning and destroying everything in their path.

In 1865, the Union army invaded and captured the Confederate capital of Richmond Virginia. Robert E. Lee, leader of the Confederacy surrendered to General Ulysses S. Grant, leader of the Union forces, on April 9, 1865. The Civil War was over and the Union was preserved.

35. What does the word secede most nearly mean?

a. To break away from

b. To accomplish

c. To join

d. To lose

36. Which of the following statements summarizes a FACT from the passage?

a. Congress declared war and then the Battle of Fort Sumter began.

b. Congress declared war after shots were fired at Fort Sumter.

c. President Lincoln was pro slavery

d. President Lincoln was at Fort Sumter with Congress

37. Which event finally led the Confederacy to surrender?

a. The battle of Gettysburg

b. The battle of Bull Run

c. The invasion of the confederate capital of Richmond

d. Sherman's March to the Sea

38. The word abolish as used in this passage most nearly means?

    a. To ban

    b. To polish

    c. To support

    d. To destroy

Questions 39 – 42 refer to the following passage.

A Day That Will Live in Infamy! Attack on Pearl Harbor

In 1941, the world was at war. The United States was trying very hard to keep itself out of the conflict. In Europe, the countries of Germany and Italy had formed an alliance to expand their land and territory. Germany had already taken over Poland, Denmark, and parts of France. They were heading next toward England and due to all the fighting in Europe, there were battles taking place as far south as North Africa, where the German and Italian armies were fighting the British.

This got even worse when the Asian nation of Japan formed an alliance with Germany and Italy. Together, the three countries called themselves, the AXIS. Now, the war was in the Pacific as well as in Europe and Northern Africa. Many Americans thought that perhaps now was the time for the United States to join with its ally, Great Britain and stop the Axis from taking over more regions of the world.

In 1941, Franklin Roosevelt was President of the United States. His fear at the time was that Japan would try to take over many countries in Asia. He did not want to see that happen, so he moved some of the United States warships that had been stationed in San Diego, to the military base at Pearl Harbor, in Honolulu, Hawaii.

Japan quietly plotted their attack. They waited until the early hours of the morning on Sunday, December 7, 1941. Then, 350 Japanese war plans began to drop bombs on the

U.S. ships at Pearl Harbor. The first bombs fell at 7:48 am and 90 minutes later, the attack was over. Pearl Harbor was decimated. 8 battleships were damaged. Eleven ships were sunk and 300 U.S. planes were destroyed. Most devastating was the loss of life 2,400 U.S. military members was killed in the attack and 1, 282 were injured.

President Roosevelt addressed the country via the radio and said "Today is a day that will live in infamy." He asked Congress to declare war on Japan. War was declared on Japan on December 8th and on Germany and Italy on December 11th. The United States had entered World War Two.

39. After reading the passage, what can we infer that the word infamy means?

    a. Famous

    b. Remembered in a good way

    c. Remembered in a bad way

    d. Easily forgotten

40. What three countries formed the Axis?

    a. Italy, England, Germany

    b. United States, England, Italy

    c. Germany, Japan, Italy

    d. Germany, Japan, United States

41. What do you think was President Roosevelt's reason for moving warships to Pearl Harbor?

    a. He feared Japan would bomb San Diego

    b. He knew Japan was going to attack Pearl Harbor

    c. He was planning to attack Japan

    d. He wanted to try to protect Asian countries from Japanese takeover

42. Why do you think Japan chose a Sunday morning at 7:48am for their attack?

    a. They knew the military slept late

    b. There is a law against bombing countries on a Sunday

    c. They wanted the attack to catch people by surprise

    d. That was the only free time they had to **attack.**

Questions 43 – 45 refer to the following passage.

What Is Mardi Gras?

Mardi Gras is fast becoming one of the South's most famous and most celebrated holidays. The word Mardi Gras comes from the French and the literal translation is "Fat Tuesday." The holiday has also been called Shrove Tuesday, due to its associations with Lent. The purpose of Mardi Gras is to celebrate and enjoy before the Lenten season of fasting and repentance begins.

What originated by the French Explorers in New Orleans, Louisiana in the 17th century is now celebrated all over the world. Panama, Italy, Belgium and Brazil all host large scale Mardi Gras celebrations, and many smaller cities and towns celebrate this fun loving Tuesday as well. Usually held in February or early March, Mardi Gras is a day of extravagance, a day for people to eat, drink and be merry, to wear costumes, masks and to dance to jazz music.

The French explorers on the Mississippi River would be in shock today if they saw the opulence of the parades and floats that grace the New Orleans streets during Mardi Gras these days. Parades in New Orleans are divided by organizations. These are more commonly known as Krewes. Being a member of a Krewe is quite a task because Krewes are responsible for overseeing the parades. Each Krewe's parade is ruled by a Mardi Gras "King and Queen." The role of the King and Queen is to "bestow" gifts on their adoring fans as the floats ride along the street. They throw doubloons, which is fake money and usually colored green, purple and gold, which are the colors of Mardi Gras. Beads in those color shades are also thrown and cups are thrown as well. Beads are by far the most popular souvenir of any Mardi Gras parade, with each spectator attempting to gather as many as possible.

43. The purpose of Mardi Gras is to

    a. Repent for a month.

    b. Celebrate in extravagant ways.

    c. Be a member of a Krewe.

    d. Explore the Mississippi.

44. From reading the passage we can infer that "Kings and Queens"

    a. Have to be members of a Krewe.

    b. Have to be French.

    c. Have to know how to speak French.

    d. Have to give away their own money.

45. Which group of people began to hold Mardi Gras celebrations?

    a. Settlers from Italy

    b. Members of Krewes

    c. French explorers

    d. Belgium explorers

Section II – Math

1. What is 1/3 of 3/4?

    a. 1/4

    b. 1/3

    c. 2/3

    d. 3/4

2. What fraction of $1500 is $75?

   a. 1/14

   b. 3/5

   c. 7/10

   d. 1/20

3. 3.14 + 2.73 + 23.7 =

   a. 28.57

   b. 30.57

   c. 29.56

   d. 29.57

4. A woman spent 15% of her income on an item and ends up with $120. What percentage of her income is left?

   a. 12%

   b. 85%

   c. 75%

   d. 95%

5. Express 0.27 + 0.33 as a fraction.

   a. 3/6

   b. 4/7

   c. 3/5

   d. 2/7

6. What is (3.13 + 7.87) X 5?

   a. 65

   b. 50

   c. 45

   d. 55

7. Reduce 2/4 X 3/4 to lowest terms.

   a. 6/12

   b. 3/8

   c. 6/16

   d. 3/4

8. 2/3 – 2/5 =

   a. 4/10

   b. 1/15

   c. 3/7

   d. 4/15

9. 2/7 + 2/3 =

   a. 12/23

   b. 5/10

   c. 20/21

   d. 6/21

10. 2/3 of 60 + 1/5 of 75 =

   a. 45

   b. 55

   c. 15

   d. 50

11. 8 is what percent of 40?

    a. 10%

    b. 15%

    c. 20%

    d. 25%

12. 9 is what percent of 36?

    a. 10%

    b. 15%

    c. 20%

    d. 25%

13. Three tenths of 90 equals:

    a. 18

    b. 45

    c. 27

    d. 36

14. .4% of 36 is

    a. 1.44

    b. .144

    c. 14.4

    d. 144

15. The physician ordered 5 mg Coumadin; 10 mg/tablet is on hand. How many tablets will you give?

    a. .5 tablets

    b. 1 tablet

    c. .75 tablets

    d. 1.5 tablets

16. The physician ordered 20 mg Tylenol/kg of body weight; on hand is 80 mg/tablet. The child weighs 12 kg. How many tablets will you give?

    a. 1 tablet

    b. 3 tablets

    c. 2 tablets

    d. 4 tablets

17. The physician ordered 20 mg Tylenol/kg of body weight; on hand is 80 mg/tablet. The child weighs 44 lb. How many tablets will you give?

    a. 5 tablets

    b. 5.5 tablets

    c. 4.5 tablets

    d. 3 tablets

18. The physician ordered 3,000 units of heparin; 5,000 U/mL is on hand. How many milliliters will you give?

    a. 0.5 ml

    b. 0.6 ml

    c. 0.75 ml

    d. 0.8 ml

19. The physician orders 60 mg Augmentin; 80 mg/mL is on hand. How many milliliters will you give?

    a. 1 ml

    b. 0.5 ml

    c. 0.75 ml

    d. 0.95 ml

20. The physician ordered 16 mg Ibuprofen/kg of body weight; on hand is 80 mg/tablet. The child weighs 15 kg. How many tablets will you give?

    a. 3 tablets

    b. 2 tablets

    c. 1 tablet

    d. 2.5 tablets

21. The physician orders 1000 mg Benbadryl liquid; 1 g/tsp is on hand. How many teaspoons will you give?

    a. .75 tsp

    b. 1.5 tsp

    c. 1 tsp

    d. 1.25 tsp

22. The physician ordered 10 units of regular insulin and 200 U/mL is on hand. How many milliliters will you give?

    a. .45 ml

    b. .75 ml

    c. .25 ml

    d. .05 ml

23. If y = 4 and x = 3, solve yx^3

    a. -108

    b. 108

    c. 27

    d. 4

24. Convert 0.007 kilograms to grams

    a. 7 grams

    b. 70 grams

    c. 0.07 grams

    d. 0.70 grams

25. Convert 16 quarts to gallons

 a. 1 gallons
 b. 8 gallons
 c. 4 gallons
 d. 4.5 gallons

26. Convert 2 teaspoons to milliliters.

 a. 4.3 milliliters
 b. 9 milliliters
 c. 9.86 milliliters
 d. 4 milliliters

27. Convert 200 meters to kilometers

 a. 50 kilometers
 b. 20 kilometers
 c. 12 kilometers
 d. 0.2 kilometers

28. Convert 72 inches to feet

 a. 12 feet
 b. 6 feet
 c. 4 feet
 d. 17 feet

29. Convert 3 yards to feet

 a. 18 feet
 b. 12 feet
 c. 9 feet
 d. 27 feet

30. Convert 45 kg. to pounds.

 a. 10 pounds
 b. 100 pounds
 c. 1,000 pounds
 d. 110 pounds

31. Convert 0.63 grams to mg.

 a. 630 g.
 b. 63 mg.
 c. 630 mg.
 d. 603 mg.

32. $5x + 3 = 7x - 1$. Find x

 a. 1/3
 b. ½
 c. 1
 d. 2

33. $5x + 2(x + 7) = 14x - 7$. Find x

 a. 1
 b. 2
 c. 3
 d. 4

34. $12t - 10 = 14t + 2$. Find t

 a. -6
 b. -4
 c. 4
 d. 6

35. $5(z + 1) = 3(z + 2) + 11$.
$Z = ?$

    a. 2

    b. 4

    c. 6

    d. 12

36. The price of a book went up from $20 to $25. What percent did the price increase?

    a. 5%

    b. 10%

    c. 20%

    d. 25%

37. The price of a book decreased from $25 to $20. What percent did the price decrease?

    a. 5%

    b. 10%

    c. 20%

    d. 25%

38. After taking several practice tests, Brian improved the results of his GRE test by 30%. Given that the first time he took the test Brian answered 150 questions correctly, how many questions did he answer correctly on the second test?

    a. 105

    b. 120

    c. 180

    d. 195

39. In local baseball team, 4 players (or 12.5% of the team) have long hair and the rest have short hair. How many short-haired players are there on the team?

    a. 24

    b. 28

    c. 32

    d. 50

40. In the time required to serve 43 customers, a server breaks 2 glasses and slips 5 times. The next day, the same server breaks 10 glasses. Assuming the number of glasses broken is proportional to the number of customers served, how many customers did she serve?

    a. 25

    b. 43

    c. 86

    d. 215

41. A square lawn has an area of 62,500 square meters. What will is the cost of building fence around it at a rate of $5.5 per meter?

    a. $4000

    b. $4500

    c. $5000

    d. $5500

42. Mr. Brown bought 5 cheese burgers, 3 drinks, and 4 fries for his family, and a cookie pack for his dog. If the price of all single items is the same at $1.30 and a 3.5% tax is added, what is the total cost of dinner for Mr. Brown?

    a. $16

    b. $16.9

    c. $17

    d. $17.5

43. The length of a rectangle is twice of its width and its area is equal to the area of a square with 12 cm. sides. What will be the perimeter of the rectangle to the nearest whole number?

    a. 36 cm

    b. 46 cm

    c. 51 cm

    d. 56 cm

44. There are 15 yellow and 35 orange balls in a basket. How many more yellow balls must be added to make the yellow balls 65%?

    a. 35

    b. 50

    c. 65

    d. 70

45. A farmer wants to plant 65,536 trees in such a way that number of rows must be equal to the number of plants in a row. How many trees should he plant in a row?

    a. 1684

    b. 1268

    c. 668

    d. 256

46. A distributor purchased 550 kilograms of potatoes for $165. He distributed these at a rate of $6.4 per 20 kilograms to 15 shops, $3.4 per 10 kilograms to 12 shops and the remainder at $1.8 per 5 kilograms. If his total distribution cost is $10, what will his profit be?

    a. $8.60

    b. $24.60

    c. $14.90

    d. $23.40

47. A farmer wants to plant trees around the outside boundaries of his rectangular field of dimensions 650 meters × 780 meters. Each tree requires 5 meters of free space all around it from the stem. How many trees can he plant?

    a. 572

    b. 568

    c. 286

    d. 282

48. 3 boys are asked to clean a surface that is 4 ft². If the surface is divided equally among the boys, how much will each clean?

    a. 1 ft 6 in²

    b. 14 in²

    c. 1 ft² in²

    d. 1 ft² 48 in²

49. How much pay does Mr. Johnson receive if he gives half of his pay to his family, $250 to his landlord, and has exactly 3/7 of his pay left over?

    a. $3600

    b. $3500

    c. $2800

    d. $1750

50. A boy has 4 red, 5 green and 2 yellow balls. He chooses two balls randomly. What is the probability that one is red and other is green?

    a. 2/11

    b. 19/22

    c. 20/121

    d. 9/11

Section III – English Grammar

1. Choose the sentence with the correct grammar.

a. Don would never have thought of that book, but you could have reminded him.

b. Don would never of thought of that book, but you could have reminded him.

c. Don would never have thought of that book, but you could of have reminded him.

d. Don would never of thought of that book, but you could of reminded him.

2. Choose the sentence with the correct grammar.

a. The man was asked to come with his daughter and her test results.

b. The man was asked to come with her daughter and her test results.

c. The man was asked to come with her daughter and our test results.

d. None of the above.

3. Choose the sentence with the proper usage.

a. They wanted to know if they may begin.

b. They wanted to know if they might begin.

c. None of the above.

4. Choose the sentence with the correct grammar.

a. Although you may not see nobody in the dark, it does not mean that nobody is there.

b. Although you may not see anyone in the dark, it does not mean that not nobody is there.

c. Although you may not see anyone in the dark, it does not mean that no one is there.

d. Although you may not see nobody in the dark, it does not mean that not nobody is there.

5. Choose the sentence with the correct grammar.

　　a. Any girl that fails the test loses their admission.

　　b. Any girl that fails the test loses our admission.

　　c. Any girl that fails the test loses her admission.

　　d. None of the above.

6. Choose the sentence with the correct grammar.

　　a.　The older children have already eat their dinner, but the baby has not yet eaten anything.

　　b.　The older children have already eaten their dinner, but the baby has not yet ate anything.

　　c.　The older children have already eaten their dinner, but the baby has not yet eaten anything.

　　d.　The older children have already eat their dinner, but the baby has not yet ate anything.

7. Choose the sentence with the correct grammar.

　　a.　If they had gone to the party, he would have gone, too.

　　b.　If they had went to the party, he would have gone, too.

　　c.　If they had gone to the party, he would have went, too.

　　d.　If they had went to the party, he would have went, too.

8. Choose the sentence with the proper usage.

　　a. He can be correct.

　　b. He could be correct.

　　c. He may be correct.

　　d. None of the above.

9. Choose the sentence with the correct grammar.

a. Everyone was asked to raise their hand.

b. Everyone was asked to raise our hand.

c. Everyone was asked to raise her hand.

d. None of the above.

10. Choose the sentence with the correct grammar.

a. Its important for you to know its official name; its called the Confederate Museum.

b. It's important for you to know it's official name; it's called the Confederate Museum.

c. It's important for you to know its official name; it's called the Confederate Museum.

d. Its important for you to know it's official name; it's called the Confederate Museum.

11. The Ford Motor Company was named for Henry Ford, _____.

a. which had founded the company.

b. who founded the company.

c. whose had founded the company.

d. whom had founded the company.

12. Thomas Edison _____ since he invented the light bulb, television, motion pictures, and phonograph.

a. has always been known as the greatest inventor

b. was always been known as the greatest inventor

c. must have had been always known as the greatest inventor

d. will had been known as the greatest inventor

13. Choose the sentence with the proper usage.

a. I will be at the office by 9 a. m.

b. I shall be at the office by 9 a. m.

c. Both of the above

d. None of the above

14. Although Joe is tall for his age, his brother Elliot is _____ of the two.

a. the tallest

b. more tallest

c. the tall

d. the taller

15. When KISS came to town, all of the tickets _____ before I could buy one.

a. will be sold out

b. had been sold out

c. were being sold out

d. was sold out

16. The rules of most sports _____ more complicated than we often realize.

a. are

b. is

c. was

d. has been

17. Choose the sentence with the correct grammar.

a. Here are the names of people whom you should contact

b. Here are the names of people who you should contact

c. Both of the above

d. None of the above.

18. The Titanic _____ mere days into its maiden voyage.

a. has already sunk

b. will already sunk

c. already sank

d. sank

19. _____ won first place in the Western Division?

a. Who

b. Whom

c. Which

d. What

20. There are now several ways to listen to music, including radio, CDs, and Mp3 files _____ you can download onto an MP3 player.

a. on which

b. who

c. whom

d. which

21. As the tallest monument in the United States, the St. Louis Arch _____.

    a. has rose to an impressive 630 feet.

    b. is risen to an impressive 630 feet.

    c. rises to an impressive 630 feet.

    d. was rose to an impressive 630 feet.

22. The tired, old woman should _____ on the sofa.

    a. lie

    b. lays

    c. laid

    d. lain

23. Did the students understand that Thanksgiving always _____ on the fourth Thursday in November?

    a. fallen

    b. falling

    c. has fell

    d. falls

24. Collecting stamps, _____ and listening to short-wave radio were Rick's main hobbies.

    a. building models,

    b. to build models,

    c. having built models,

    d. build models,

25. Choose the sentence with the correct usage.

a. The ceremony had an emotional effect on the groom, but the bride was not affected.

b. The ceremony had an emotional affect on the groom, but the bride was not affected.

c. The ceremony had an emotional effect on the groom, but the bride was not effected.

d. The ceremony had an emotional affect on the groom, but the bride was not affected.

26. Choose the sentence with the correct usage.

a. Anna was taller then Luis, but then he grew four inches in three months.

b. Anna was taller then Luis, but than he grew four inches in three months.

c. Anna was taller than Luis, but than he grew four inches in three months.

d. Anna was taller than Luis, but then he grew four inches in three months.

27. Choose the sentence with the correct usage.

a. Their second home is in Boca Raton, but there not their for most of the year.

b. They're second home is in Boca Raton, but they're not there for most of the year.

c. Their second home is in Boca Raton, but they're not there for most of the year.

d. There second home is in Boca Raton, but they're not there for most of the year.

28. Choose the sentence with the proper usage.

a. He ought to be back by now.

b. He ought be back by now.

c. He ought come back by now.

d. None of the above.

29. Choose the sentence with the correct grammar.

a. Mark and Peter have talked to each other.

b. Mark and Peter have talked to one another.

c. Both of the above.

d. None of the above.

30. Choose the sentence with the correct usage.

a. You're classes are on the west side of campus, but you're living on the east side.

b. Your classes are on the west side of campus, but your living on the east side.

c. Your classes are on the west side of campus, but you're living on the east side.

d. You're classes are on the west side of campus, but you're living on the east side.

31. Choose the sentence with the correct usage.

a. Disease is highly prevalent in poorer nations; the most dominant disease is malaria.

b. Disease are highly prevalent in poorer nations; the most dominant disease is malaria.

c. Disease is highly prevalent in poorer nations; the most dominant disease are malaria.

d. Disease are highly prevalent in poorer nations; the most dominant disease are malaria.

32. Choose the sentence with the correct usage.

a. Although I would prefer to have dog, I actually own a cat.

b. Although I would prefer to have a dog, I actually own cat.

c. Although I would prefer to have a dog, I actually own a cat.

d. Although I would prefer to have dog, I actually own cat.

33. Choose the sentence with the correct usage.

a. The principal of the school lived by one principle: always do your best.

b. The principle of the school lived by one principle: always do your best.

c. The principal of the school lived by one principal: always do your best.

d. The principle of the school lived by one principal: always do your best.

34. Choose the sentence with the correct usage.

a. Even with an speed limit sign clearly posted, an inattentive driver may drive too fast.

b. Even with a speed limit sign clearly posted, a inattentive driver may drive too fast.

c. Even with an speed limit sign clearly posted, a inattentive driver may drive too fast.

d. Even with a speed limit sign clearly posted, an inattentive driver may drive too fast.

35. Choose the sentence with the correct usage.

a. Except for the roses, she did not accept John's frequent gifts.

b. Accept for the roses, she did not except John's frequent gifts.

c. Accept for the roses, she did not accept John's frequent gifts.

d. Except for the roses, she did not except John's frequent gifts.

36. Choose the sentence with the correct usage.

a. Although he continued to advise me, I no longer took his advice.

b. Although he continued to advice me, I no longer took his advise.

c. Although he continued to advise me, I no longer took his advise.

d. Although he continued to advice me, I no longer took his advise.

37. Choose the sentence with the correct usage.

a. To adopt to the climate, we had to adopt a different style of clothing.

b. To adapt to the climate, we had to adapt a different style of clothing.

c. To adapt to the climate, we had to adopt a different style of clothing.

d. To adapt to the climate, we had to adapt a different style of clothing.

38. Choose the sentence with the correct usage.

a. When he's between friends, Robert seems confident, but between you and me, he is really very shy.

b. When he's among friends, Robert seems confident, but among you and me, he is really very shy.

c. When he's between friends, Robert seems confident, but among you and me, he is really very shy.

d. When he's among friends, Robert seems confident, but between you and me, he is really very shy.

39. Choose the sentence with the correct usage.

a. I will be finished at ten in the morning, and will be arriving at home at about 6:30.

b. I will be finished at about ten in the morning, and will be arriving at home at 6:30.

c. I will be finished at about ten in the morning, and will be arriving at home at about 6:30.

d. I will be finished at ten in the morning, and will be arriving at home at 6:30.

40. Choose the sentence with the correct usage.

a. Beside the red curtains and pillows, there was a red rug beside the couch.

b. Besides the red curtains and pillows, there was a red rug beside the couch.

c. Besides the red curtains and pillows, there was a red rug besides the couch.

d. Beside the red curtains and pillows, there was a red rug besides the couch.

41. Choose the sentence with the correct usage.

a. Although John can swim very well, the lifeguard may not allow him to swim in the pool.

b. Although John may swim very well, the lifeguard may not allow him to swim in the pool.

c. Although John can swim very well, the lifeguard cannot allow him to swim in the pool.

d. Although John may swim very well, the lifeguard may not allow him to swim in the pool.

42. Choose the sentence with the correct usage.

a. Her continuous absences caused a continual disruption at the office.

b. Her continual absences caused a continuous disruption at the office.

c. Her continual absences caused a continual disruption at the office.

d. Her continuous absences caused a continuous disruption at the office.

43. Choose the sentence with the correct usage.

a. During the famine, the Irish people had to emigrate to other countries; many of them immigrated to the United States.

b. During the famine, the Irish people had to immigrate to other countries; many of them immigrated to the United States.

c. During the famine, the Irish people had to emigrate to other countries; many of them emigrated to the United States.

d. During the famine, the Irish people had to immigrate to other countries; many of them emigrated to the United States.

44. Choose the sentence with the correct usage.

a. His home was farther than we expected; farther, the roads were very bad.

b. His home was farther than we expected; further, the roads were very bad.

c. His home was further than we expected; further, the roads were very bad.

d. His home was further than we expected; farther, the roads were very bad.

45. Choose the sentence with the correct usage.

a. The volunteers brought groceries and toys to the homeless shelter; the latter were given to the staff, while the former were given directly to the children.

b. The volunteers brought groceries and toys to the homeless shelter; the former was given to the staff, while the latter was given directly to the children.

c. The volunteers brought groceries and toys to the homeless shelter; the groceries were given to the staff, while the former was given directly to the children.

d. The volunteers brought groceries and toys to the homeless shelter; the latter was given to the staff, while the groceries were given directly to the children.

46. Choose the sentence with the correct usage.

a. Vegetables are a healthy food; eating them can make you more healthful.

b. Vegetables are a healthful food; eating them can make you more healthful.

c. Vegetables are a healthy food; eating them can make you more healthy.

d. Vegetables are a healthful food; eating them can make you more healthy.

47. Choose the sentence with the correct usage.

a. After you lay the books on the counter, you may lay down for a nap.

b. After you lie the books on the counter, you may lay down for a nap.

c. After you lay the books on the counter, you may lie down for a nap.

d. After you lay the books on the counter, you may lay down for a nap.

48. Choose the sentence with the correct usage.

a. After you lay the books on the counter, you may lay down for a nap.

b. After you lie the books on the counter, you may lay down for a nap.

c. After you lay the books on the counter, you may lie down for a nap.

d. After you lay the books on the counter, you may lay down for a nap.

49. Choose the sentence with the correct usage.

a. Once the chickens had layed their eggs, they lay on their nests to hatch them.

b. Once the chickens had lay their eggs, they lay on their nests to hatch them.

c. Once the chickens had laid their eggs, they lay on their nests to hatch them.

d. Once the chickens had laid their eggs, they laid on their nests to hatch them.

50. Choose the sentence with the correct usage.

a. Mrs. Foster taught me many things, but I learned the most from Mr. Wallace.

b. Mrs. Foster learned me many things, but I was taught the most by Mr. Wallace.

c. Mrs. Foster learned me many things, but I learned the most from Mr. Wallace.

d. Mrs. Foster taught me many things, but I was learned the most from Mr. Wallace.

Section IV – Vocabulary

1. Choose a verb that means fearless or invulnerable to intimidation and fear.

    a. Feeble

    b. Strongest

    c. Dauntless

    d. Super

2. Choose a word that means the same as the underlined word.

I see the differences when they are placed side-by-side and <u>juxtaposed.</u>

    a. Compared

    b. Eliminated

    c. Overturned

    d. Exonerated

3. Choose the best definition of regicide.

    a. v. To endow or furnish with requisite ability, character, knowledge and skill

    b. n. killing of a king

    c. adj. Disposed to seize by violence or by unlawful or greedy methods

    d. v. To refresh after labor

4. Choose the best definition of pernicious.

    a. Deadly

    b. Infectious

    c. Common

    d. Rare

5. Fill in the blank.

After she received her influenza vaccination, Nan thought that she was _____ to the common cold.

    a. Immune

    b. Susceptible

    c. Vulnerable

    d. At risk

6. Choose a word that means the same as the underlined word.

She performed the gymnastics and stretches so well! I have never seen anyone so <u>nimble</u>.

    a. Awkward

    b. Agile

    c. Quick

    d. Taut

7. Choose a word that means the same as the underlined word.

Are there any more <u>queries</u>? We have already had so many questions today.

    a. Questions

    b. Commands

    c. Obfuscations

    d. Paradoxes

8. Choose a verb that means to remove a leader or high official from position.

    a. Sack

    b. Suspend

    c. Depose

    d. Dropped

9. Choose the best definition of pedestrian.

    a. Rare

    b. Often

    c. Walking or Running

    d. Commonplace

10. Choose the best definition of petulant.

    a. Patient

    b. Childish

    c. Impatient

    d. Mature

11. Fill in the blank.

Paul's rose bushes were being destroyed by Japanese beetles, so he invested in a good _____.

    a. Fungicide

    b. Fertilizer

    c. Sprinkler

    d. Pesticide

12. Choose the best definition of salient.

    a. v. To make light by fermentation, as dough

    b. adj. Not stringent or energetic

    c. adj. negligible

    d. adj. worthy of note or relevant

13. Choose the best definition of sedentary.

a. n. A morbid condition, due to obstructed excretion of bile or characterized by yellowing of the skin

b. adj. not moving or sitting at a place

c. v. To wander from place to place

d. n. Perplexity

14. Fill in the blank.

The last time that the crops failed, the entire nation experienced months of _____.

a. Famine

b. Harvest

c. Plenitude

d. Disease

15. Choose the best definition of stint.

a. Thrifty

b. Annoyed

c. Dislike

d. Insult

16. Choose the best definition of precipitate.

a. To rain

b. To throw down

c. To throw up

d. to snow

17. Choose the verb that means to build up or strengthen in relation to morals or religion.

   a. Sanctify

   b. Amplify

   c. Edify

   d. Wry

18. Choose the noun that means exit or way out.

   a. Door-jamb

   b. Egress

   c. Regress

   d. Furtherance

19. Choose the best definition of the underlined word.

The tide was in this morning but now it is starting to recede.

   a. Go out

   b. Flow

   c. Swell

   d. Come in

20. Choose the word that means private, personal.

   a. Confidential

   b. Hysteric

   c. Simplistic

   d. Promissory

21. Choose the best definition of the underlined word.

I don't think that will make it any better - it is just going to <u>aggravate</u> the situation.

- a. Worsen
- b. Precipitate
- c. Elongate
- d. None of the above

22. Choose the best definition of the underlined word.

I didn't think this was her first appearance, but it is her <u>debut</u>.

- a. Exit
- b. Introduction
- c. Curtain Call
- d. Resignation

23. Fill in the blank.

Because of a pituitary dysfunction, Karl lacked the necessary _____ to grow as tall as his father.

- a. Glands
- b. Hormones
- c. Vitamins
- d. Testosterone

24. Choose the best definition of importune.

- a. To find an opportunity
- b. To ask all the time
- c. Cannot find an opportunity
- d. None of the above

25. Choose the best definition of sedulous.

    a. n. The support on or against which a lever rests

    b. adj. constant steady pursuit

    c. v. To oppose with an equal force

    d. n. The branch of medical science that relates to improving health

26. Choose the best definition of tincture.

    a. n. alcoholic drink with plant extract used for medicine

    b. n. An artificial trance-sleep

    c. n. a special medicinal drink made by mixing water with plant extracts

    d. adj. the point of puncture

27. Choose the noun that means serious criminal offence that is punishable by death or imprisonment above a year

    a. Trespass

    b. Hampers

    c. Felony

    d. Obligatory

28. Choose the best meaning of the underlined word.

His library is enormous. I didn't realize he was such a <u>bibliophile</u>.

    a. Book lover

    b. Audiophile

    c. Bibliophobe

    d. Audiophobe

29. Fill in the blank.

When Mr. Davis returned from southern Asia, he told us about the _____ that sometimes swept the area, bringing torrential rain.

    a. Monsoons

    b. Hurricanes

    c. Blizzards

    d. Floods

30. Choose the best definition of volatile.

    a. Not explosive

    b. Catches fire easily

    c. Does not catch fire

    d. Explosive

31. Choose the word that means the same as plaintive.

    a. Happy

    b. Mournful

    c. Faint

    d. Plain

32. What is the best definition of truism?

    a. n. A comparison which directs the mind to the representative object itself

    b. n. self evident or clear obvious truth

    c. n. a statement that is true but that can hardly be proved

    d. n. false statements

33. Choose the verb that means to encourage or incite troublesome acts.

    a. Comment

    b. Foment

    c. Integument

    d. Atonement

34. Choose the adjective that means dignified, solemn that is appropriate for a funeral.

    a. Funereal

    b. Prediction

    c. Wailing

    d. Vociferous

35. Choose the best definition for the underlined word.

I thought they were being very discreet, but they were, in fact, very <u>flagrant</u>.

    a. Obvious

    b. Secretive

    c. Hidden

    d. Subtle

36. Fill in the blank.

Is it true that _____ always grows on the north side of trees?

    a. Lichens

    b. Moss

    c. Ferns

    d. Ground cover

37. Choose the best definition of nexus.

a. A connection

b. A telephone switch

c. Part of a computer

d. None of the above.

38. Choose the best definition of zealot.

a. n. a person who is very passionate and fanatic about his specific objectives or beliefs

b. n. The property or state of allowing the passage of light

c. adj. Existing for a short time only

d. n. An interpreter

39. Choose the best definition of vertigo.

a. n. Hard or agonizing labor

b. n. dizziness

c. n. a spicy shrub found on the mountain plains of East Africa

d. adj. pain caused by falling from a high height

40. Choose the best definition of trenchant.

a. adj. Vigorous or incisive in expression or style.

b. n. A specific capability of feeling or emotion

c. n. A word having the same or almost the same meaning as some other

d. n. a military jacket that is also bullet proof

41. Choose the noun that means warmth and kindness of disposition.

   a. Seethe

   b. Geniality

   c. Desists

   d. Predicate

42. He goes for coffee everyday. It is his habitual start to the day.

   a. Customary

   b. Rare

   c. Unchanging

   d. Unusual

43. Choose the best definition for the underlined word.

She is just crazy about Britney Spears. She <u>idolizes</u> her a little too much I think.

   a. Fears

   b. Worships

   c. Rejects

   d. Refutes

44. Choose the best definition of osculate.

   a. v. to rotate anti clockwise

   b. v. to rescue

   c. v. to kiss or related to kissing

   d. v. to break into little pieces

45. Choose the best definition of conjoin.

   a. A connection

   b. To marry

   c. Weld together

   d. To join together

46. Choose the best definition of petrify.

    a. Turn into a fossil

    b. Turn to stone

    c. Turn into wood

    d. Turn into glass

47. Fill in the blank.

You can _____ some fires by covering them with dirt, while others require foam or water.

    a. Extinguish

    b. Distinguish

    c. Ignite

    d. Lessen

48. Fill in the blank.

Through the use of powerful fans that circulate the heat over the food, _____ ovens work very efficiently.

    a. Microwave

    b. Broiler

    c. Convection

    d. Pressure

49. Select the word that means the same as the underlined word.

She has been to some very dangerous places. She is an <u>intrepid</u> explorer.

    a. Brave

    b. Timid

    c. Timorous

    d. Cowardly

50. Choose the verb that means to encourage, stimulate or incite and provoke.

    a. Push

    b. Force

    c. Threaten

    d. Goad

Section V – Science

1. A motorcycle travelling 90 mph accelerates to pass a truck. Five seconds later the car is going 120 mph. Calculate the motorcycles' acceleration.

    a. 5 mph/second^2

    b. 10 mph/second^2

    c. 15 mph/second^2

    d. 20 mph/second^2

2. Which of the following disciplines have a close relationship with cell biology?

    a. Genetics

    b. Genealogy

    . c. Paleontology

    d. Archaeology

3. A solution with a pH value of greater than 7 is

    a. Base

    b. Acid

    c. Neutral

    d. None of the above

4. Ohm's law states

a. The voltage across a resistor is not equal to the product of the resistance and the current flowing through it.

b. The voltage across a resistor is equal to the product of the resistance and the current flowing through it.

c. The voltage across a resistor is greater than the product of the resistance.

d. The voltage across a resistor is equal to the current flowing through it.

5. Which statement below regarding Eukaryotic and prokaryotic cells is correct?

a. Both are organelles

b. Eukaryotic are not organelles

c. Both have DNA

d. Both have single membrane compartments

6. Electricity is a general term encompassing a variety of phenomena resulting from the presence and flow of electric charge. Which of the following statements about electricity is/are true?

a. Electrically charged matter is influenced by, and produces, electromagnetic fields.

b. Electric current is a movement or flow of electrically charged particles.

c. Electric potential is a fundamental interaction between the magnetic field and the presence and motion of an electric charge.

d. An influence produced by an electric charge on other charges in its vicinity is an electric field.

7. Which of these is not a process involved in cellular biology?

    a. Active transport

    b. Adhesion

    c. Subversion

    d. Cell signaling

8. When we say that important traits for scientific classification are homologous, "homologous" means

    a. Being shared among two or more animals with the same parent.

    b. Being coincidentally shared by two totally different creatures.

    c. Being inherited by the organisms' common ancestors.

    d. Mutating beyond all reasonable expectations.

9. The manner in which instructions for building proteins, the basic structural molecules of living material are written in the DNA, is

    a. Genotypic assignment

    b. Chromosome pattern

    c. Genetic code

    d. Genetic fingerprinting

10. A _____ is a unit of inherited material, encoded by a strand of DNA and transcribed by RNA.

    a. Allele

    b. Phenotype

    c. Gene

    d. Genotype

11. A runner can sprint 6 meters per second. How far will she travel in 2 minutes?

    a. 600 meters

    b. 720 meters

    c. 760 meters

    d. 800 meters

12. Which of these is not an area studied in cell biology?

    a. Cells physiological properties

    b. Cell structure

    c. Cell life cycle

    d. Cellular scientists' biographies

13. Why is detection of pathogens complicated?

    a. They evolve so quickly

    b. They die so quickly

    c. They are invisible

    d. They multiply so quickly

14. Calculate the molarity of a sugar solution if 4 liters of the solution contains 8 moles of sugar?

    a. 0.5 M

    b. 8 M

    c. 2 M

    d. 80 M

15. Which of the following is/are not included in Ohm's Law?

a. Ohm's Law defines the relationships between (P) power, (E) voltage, (I) current, and (R) resistance.

b. One ohm is the resistance value through which one volt will maintain a current of one ampere.

c. Using Ohm's Law, voltage is determined using V = IR, with I equaling current and R equaling resistance.

d. An ohm (Ω) is a unit of electrical voltage.

16. How many elements are represented on the modern periodic table?

a. 122 elements

b. 99 elements

c. 102 elements

d. 118 elements

17. Which, if any, of the following statements are false?

a. A mutation is a permanent change in the DNA sequence of a gene.

b. Mutations in a gene's DNA sequence can alter the amino acid sequence of the protein encoded by the gene.

c. Mutations in DNA sequences usually occur spontaneously.

d. Mutations in DNA sequences can caused by exposure to environmental agents such as sunshine.

18. Three cars are travelling down an even road at a velocity of 110 m/s, calculate the car with the highest momentum if they are all moving at the same speed, but the first car weighs 2500 kg, second car weighs 2650 kg and third car weighs 2009 kg?

    a. First car

    b. Second car

    d. Third car

    d. All have same momentum

19. Starting with the weakest, arrange the fundamental forces of nature in order of strength.

    a. Gravity, Weak Nuclear Force, Electromagnetic Force, Strong Nuclear Force

    b. Weak Nuclear Force, Gravity, Electromagnetic Force, Strong Nuclear Force

    c. Strong Nuclear Force, Weak Nuclear Force, Electromagnetic Force, Gravity

    d. Gravity, Strong Nuclear Force, Weak Nuclear Force, Electromagnetic Force

20. What are electrons?

    a. Subatomic particles that carry a negative charge

    b. Subatomic particles that carry a positive charge

    c. Subatomic particles that carry both a negative and positive charge

    d. None of the above

21. Cell culture is defined as

a. The technique for growing cells independent of a living organism within the confines of a laboratory.

b. The process of killing cells through use of lasers.

c. The method of creating cellular communities.

d. A method for localizing proteins in tissue slices.

22. _____, which refers to the repeatability of measurement, does not require knowledge of the correct or true value.

a. Precision

b. Value

c. Certainty

d. Accuracy

23. Describe a conductor.

a. A conductor contains a moving electrical charge.

b. A conductor will move an electrical charge depending on the size.

c. A conductor contains an electrical charge which will move when an electric potential difference is applied.

d. None of the above

24. Describe the periodic table.

a. The periodic table is a tabular display of the chemical compounds organized on the basis of their atomic numbers, electron configurations, and recurring chemical properties.

b. The periodic table is a tabular display of the chemical elements, organized on the basis of their atomic numbers, electron configurations, and recurring chemical properties.

c. The periodic table is a tabular display of the chemical subatomic particles, organized on the basis of their atomic numbers, electron configurations, and recurring chemical properties.

d. None of the above.

25. The scientific discipline that studies the physiological aspects, structures, life cycles and division of cells is called _____.

    a. Physiology

    b. Cell science

    c. Biochemistry

    d. Cell biology

26. What is the minimum amount of energy required to remove an electron from an atom or ion in the gas phase?

    a. Ionization energy

    b. Valence energy

    c. Atomic energy

    d. Ionic energy

27. In a redox reaction, the number of electrons lost is

    a. Less than the number of electrons gained

    b. More than the number of electrons gained

    c. Equal to the number of electrons gained

    d. None of the above

28. In terms of the scientific method, the term _____ refers to the act of noticing or perceiving something and/or recording a fact or occurrence.

    a. Observation

    b. Diligence

    c. Perception

    d. Control

29. The _____ Theory defines acids and bases in terms of the electron-pair concept; according to its definition, an acid is an electron-pair acceptor, and a base is an electron-pair donor.

    a. Arrhenius

    b. Lewis

    c. Clark

    d. Brønstead-Lowry

30. What is the molarity of a solution containing 5 moles of solute in 250 milliliters of solution?

    a. 20 M

    b. 15 M

    c. 0.104 M

    d. 1.25 M

31. The property of a conductor that restricts its internal flow of electrons is:

    a. Friction

    b. Power

    c. Current

    d. Resistance

32. Describe bacteria.

    a. Prokaryotic microorganisms that are usually just a few micrometres long.

    b. A single-celled organism.

    c. A virus.

    d. Three or more molecules clumped together.

33. What is the difference, of any, between kinetic energy and potential energy?

a. Kinetic energy is the energy of a body that results from heat while potential energy is the energy possessed by an object that is chilled.

b. Kinetic energy is the energy of a body that results from motion while potential energy is the energy possessed by an object by virtue of its position or state, e.g., as in a compressed spring.

c. There is no difference between kinetic and potential energy; all energy is the same.

d. Potential energy is the energy of a body that results from motion while kinetic energy is the energy possessed by an object by virtue of its position or state, e.g., as in a compressed spring.

34. A rocket releases a satellite into orbit around Earth. The satellite travels at 2000 m/s in 25 seconds. What is the acceleration?

a. 60 m/sec^2

b. 80 m/sec^2

c. 100 m/sec^2

d. 120 m/sec^2

35. Name the four states in which matter exists.

a. Concrete, liquid, gas, and plasma

b. Solid, fluid, gas, and plasma

c. Solid, , vapor, and plasma

d. Solid, liquid, gas, and plasma

36. Which one of the following best describes the function of a cell membrane?

a. It controls the substances entering and leaving the cell.

b. It keeps the cell in shape.

c. It controls the substances entering the cell.

d. It supports the cell structures

37. Describe electric current.

a. Electric current is the flow of voltage

b. Electric current is the movement of negative ions.

c. Electric current is the flow of electric charge through a medium.

d. None of the above

38. Which of the following is not a typical shape for a bacterium?

a. Rod

b. Spiral

c. Sphere

d. Cube

39. What is usually the result when acid reacts with most of the metals?

a. Carbon dioxide

b. Oxygen gas

c. Nitrogen gas

d. Hydrogen gas

40. Which of these is not a rank within the area of classification or taxonomy?

   a. Species

   b. Family

   c. Genus

   d. Relative position

41. Which of the following statements about the periodic table of the elements is true?

   a. On the periodic table, the elements are arranged according to their atomic mass.

   b. The way in which the elements are arranged allows for predictions to made about their behavior.

   c. The vertical columns of the table are called rows.

   d. The horizontal rows of the table are called groups.

42. The scientific term _____ refers to a practical test designed with the intention that its results be relevant to a particular theory or set of theories.

   a. Procedure

   b. Variable

   c. Hypothesis

   d. Experiment

43. Substances that deactivate catalysts are called

   a. Inhibitors

   b. Catalytic poisons

   c. Positive catalysts

   d. None of the above

44. What is the force per unit area exerted against a surface by the weight of air above that surface in the Earth's atmosphere?

   a. Gravitational force

   b. Atmospheric pressure

   c. Barometric density

   d. Aneroid pressure

45. Describe kinetic energy.

   a. Kinetic energy is the energy an object possesses due to its mass.

   b. Kinetic energy is the energy an object possesses due to its motion.

   c. Kinetic energy is the energy an object possesses due to its chemical properties.

   d. Kinetic energy is the stored energy an object possesses.

46. Another term for biological classification is:

   a. Darwinian classification

   b. Animal classification

   c. Molecular classification

   d. Scientific classification

47. When do oxidation and reduction reactions occur?

   a. One after the other

   b. In separate reactions

   c. On the product side of the reaction

   d. Simultaneously

48. What type of gene is not expressed as a trait unless inherited by both parents?

   a. Principal gene

   b. Latent gene

   c. Recessive gene

   d. Dominant gene

49. A _____ _____ is an approximation or simulation of a real system that omits all but the most essential variables of the system.

   a. Scientific method

   b. Independent variable

   c. Control group

   d. Scientific model

50. A proton is:

   a. A subatomic particle that forms part of the nucleus on an atom.

   b. The nucleus of an atom.

   c. An atomic particle that forms part of the nucleus on an atom.

   d. A microscopic particle that forms part of the nucleus on an atom.

51. Neutrons are necessary within an atomic nucleus because

   a. They bind with protons via nuclear force

   b. They bind with nuclei via nuclear force

   c. They bind with protons via electromagnetic force

   d. They bind with nuclei via electromagnetic force

52. How do atoms of different elements combine to form chemical mixtures?

a. Atoms of different elements combine in simple whole-number ratios to form chemical compounds.

b. Atoms of different components combine in simple fractional ratios to form chemical compounds.

c. Atoms of the same element combine in simple whole-number ratios to form chemical compounds.

d. Atoms of different elements combine in simple whole-number ratios to form chemical mixtures.

53. Which of the following statements is false?

a. Most enzymes are proteins

b. Enzymes are catalysts

c. Most enzymes are inorganic

d. Enzymes are large biological molecules

54. _____ are compounds that contain hydrogen, can dissolve in water to release hydrogen ions into solution, and, in an aqueous solution, can conduct electricity.

a. Caustics

b. Bases

c. Acids

d. Salts

55. Find the momentum of a round stone weighing 12.05 kg rolling down a hill at 8 m/s.

a. 95 kg m/sec down the hill.

b. 96.4 kg m/sec down the hill.

c. 100 kg m/sec down the hill.

d. 90 kg m/sec down the hill.

56. Which of the following statements about non-metals are false?

a. A non-metal is a substance that conducts heat and electricity poorly.

b. The majority of the known chemical elements are non-metals.

c. A non-metal is brittle or waxy or gaseous.

d. None of the statements are false.

57. What is the name of the discipline that studies bacteria?

a. Bacteriography

b. Bacteriology

c. Bacteriepathy

d. Bacterioscopy

58. What are the basic structural units of nucleic acids (DNA or RNA) whose sequence determines individual hereditary characteristics?

a. Gene

b. Nucleotide

c. Phosphate

d. Nitrogen base

59. Which of these statements about light energy is/are true?

a. Light consists of electromagnetic waves in the visible range.

b. The fundamental particle or quantum of light is a photon.

c. A and B are true.

d. None of the statements are true.

60. List the classifications of organisms in order of size.

a. Genus, Kingdom, Phylum/division, Class, Order, and Family Species

b. Order, Kingdom, Phylum/division, Genus, Class, and Family Species

c. Genus, Kingdom, Phylum/division, Class, Order, and Family Species

d. Kingdom ,Genus, Phylum/division, Class, Order, and Family Species

e. Family species, Order, Class, Phylum/division, Kingdom, and Genus

61. Explain chemical bonds.

a. Chemical bonds are attractions between atoms that form chemical substances containing two or more atoms.

b. Chemical bonds are attractions between protons that form chemical elements containing two or more atoms.

c. Chemical bonds are two or more atoms that form chemical substances.

d. None of the above

62. The number of protons in the nucleus of an atom is the

a. Atomic mass.

b. Atomic weight.

c. Atomic number.

d. None of the above.

63. The molarity of an aqueous solution of CaCl is defined as the

    a. moles of CaCl per milliliter of solution

    b. grams of CaCl per liter of water

    c. grams of CaCl per milliliter of solution

    d. moles of CaCl per liter of solution

64. An electron is:

    a. A tiny particle with a negative charge.

    b. A tiny particle with a positive charge.

    c. A tiny particle with a negative charge that orbits a nucleus.

    d. A tiny particle with a positive charge that orbits an atom.

65. What law states that, in a chemical change, energy can be neither created nor destroyed, but only changed from one form to another?

    a. The Law of the Preservation of Matter

    b. The Law of the Conservation of Energy

    c. The Law of the Conservation of Energy

    d. The Law of the Conservation of Energy

66. What is the simplest unit of any compound?

    a. Atom

    b. Proton

    c. Molecule

    d. Compound

67. Sex chromosomes are designated as being "X" or "Y" chromosomes. In terms of sex chromosomes, what differences exist between males and females?

a. Females have two X chromosomes and males have one X chromosome and one Y chromosome.

b. Females have one X chromosome, and males have one X chromosome and one Y chromosome.

c. Females have one Y chromosome, while males have one X chromosome.

d. Females have one X chromosome and one Y chromosome, and males have two X chromosomes.

68. A biofilm is

a. A dense aggregation of bacteria attached to surfaces.

b. A type of bacteria which causes disease.

c. A cluster of bacteria which is healthy to consume.

d. Bacteria which aids in digestion.

69. Identify the chemical properties of water.

a. Water has two hydrogen atoms covalently bonded to one oxygen atom.

b. Water has two oxygen atoms covalently bonded to one hydrogen atom.

c. Water has two hydrogen atoms polar covalently bonded to one oxygen atom.

d. Water has two oxygen atoms polar covalently bonded to one hydrogen atom.

70. What unit is electrical resistance measured?

a. Ohms

b. Volts

c. Amps

d. None of the above

71. Calculate the molarity of 2.5 liters of a lithium fluoride, LiF solution that contains 52 grams of LiF.

(Gram-formula - atomic mass = 26 grams/mole)

    a. 0.8 M

    b. 1.5 M

    c. 0.5 mol

    d. 2 mol

72. In physics, _____ is the force that opposes the relative motion of two bodies in contact.

    a. Resistance

    b. Abrasiveness

    c. Friction

    d. Antagonism

73. What is the difference between anabolism and catabolism?

    a. Anabolism is the series of chemical reactions resulting in the synthesis of inorganic compounds, and catabolism is a series of chemical reactions that break down larger molecules.

    b. Anabolism is the series of chemical reactions resulting in the synthesis of organic compounds, and catabolism is a series of chemical reactions that combine larger molecules.

    c. Catabolism is the series of chemical reactions resulting in the synthesis of organic compounds, and anabolism is a series of chemical reactions that break down larger molecules.

    d. Anabolism is the series of chemical reactions resulting in the synthesis of organic compounds, and catabolism is a series of chemical reactions that break down larger molecules.

74. What results when acid reacts with a base?

    a. A weak acid

    b. A weak base

    c. A salt and water

    d. Hydrogen

75. What is a reaction where an element gains electrons is known as?

    a. Reduction

    b. Oxidation

    c. Sublimation

    d. Condensation

Section VI - Anatomy and Physiology

1. The quadrant that is largely responsible for digestion is _____.

    a. Left Upper

    b. Right Upper

    c. Right Left

    d. Left Lower

2. Human homeostasis is the ability of the body to regulate its _____ in response to fluctuations in the environment outside the body.

    a. Inner environment

    b. Outer environment

    c. Temperature

    d. Metabolism

3. An important function of epithelial tissue is

a. Strengthen the muscles.

b. Acting as a protective barrier for the human body.

c. Protect the nerves.

d. Nonexistent; it has been found to have no known function.

4. The bodily organ system which protects the person's body from damage is the _____ system.

a. Circulatory

b. Musculoskeletal

c. Integumentary

d. Digestive

5. Another primary purpose of the musculoskeletal system is

a. Moving oxygen

b. Cleansing the blood stream

c. Relaxing the mind

d. Providing form for the body

6. What are examples of nutrients passed along via the circulatory system?

a. Citric acids

b. Amino acids

c. Proteins

d. Nuclei

7. Which of the following is an example of an important component of the respiratory system?

a. The cornea

b. The lungs

c. The kidneys

d. The stomach

8. How does the immune system fight off disease?

a. By identifying and killing tumor cells and pathogens.

b. By creating new blood cells that fight disease.

c. By expelling infection through the blood stream.

d. By giving you energy to resist disease infections.

9. What is the primary purpose of the digestive system?

a. To expel food and liquids from the body.

b. To absorb oxygen from food.

c. To help circulate blood throughout the body.

d. To convert food into a form that can provide nourishment for the body.

10. What is mostly true of urine?

a. It's mostly comprised of healthy vitamins and nutrients.

b. It's mostly comprised of waste material after the body has taken the nutrients from food and absorbed the water it needs.

c. It's mostly useless in the body.

d. It's mostly carbohydrates.

11. The gallbladder is located in the

a. RUQ

b. LUQ

c. LLQ

d. RLQ

12. The lymphatic system is defined as the system which

a. Carries a clear liquid ("lymph") toward the heart.

b. Carries a clear liquid ("lymph") out through the bowels.

c. Heals the lymph nodes.

d. Cleanses the blood stream of bacteria.

13. Which organ of the body acts as a biological filter of blood?

a. The spleen

b. Bone marrow

c. The liver

d. The heart

14. The body organ that is NOT located within the Right Upper Quadrant is

a. Liver

b. Gall Bladder

c. Duodenum

d. Sigmoid colon

15. An example of a person whose metabolism has lowered is

a. A woman who is in her teens and quite athletic.

b. A man who is past 30 and whose body is losing muscle.

c. A man who is past 30 and works out daily.

d. A man who is past 30 and eats a low-fat diet.

16. Muscle tissue has the ability to _____, bringing out movement and the ability to work.

a. Divide and conquer

b. Replicate at will

c. Relax and contract

d. Sleep

17. How many layers of skin are contained within the human integumentary system (skin)?

a. One

b. Two

c. Three

d. Four

18. What is cartilage?

a. A flexible, connective tissue that keeps bones from rubbing against each other

b. The material that comprises the brain

c. A part of human blood responsible for fighting infection

d. Another name for the femur

19. What are the main components of the circulatory system?

a. The heart, veins and blood vessels

b. The heart, brain, and ears

c. The nose, throat and ears

d. The lungs, stomach, and kidneys

20. The exchange of oxygen for carbon dioxide takes place in the alveolar area of

a. The throat

b. The ears

c. The appendix

d. The lungs

21. Detection of pathogens can be complicated because

a. They evolve so quickly

b. They die so quickly

c. They are invisible

d. They multiply so quickly

22. Which of these is not an example of a function of the stomach in digestion?

a. Storing food

b. Cleansing food of impurities

c. Mixing food with digestive juices

d. Transferring food into the intestines

23. What is the name of the waste removed from the body through urine?

a. Urea

b. Urinalysis

c. Feces

d. Fat

24. An example of an organ that plays a big role in the lymphatic system is

a. The spine

b. The kidney

c. The spleen

d. The liver

25. What controls reflex action?

a. The sympathetic nervous system

b. The parasympathetic nervous system.

c. The central nervous system

d. The sensory nerves

Answer Key

Section 1 – Reading Comprehension

1. B
We can infer from this passage that sickness from an infectious disease can be easily transmitted from one person to another.

From the passage, "Infectious pathologies are also called communicable diseases or transmissible diseases, due to their potential of transmission from one person or species to another by a replicating agent (as opposed to a toxin)."

2. A
Two other names for infectious pathologies are communicable diseases and transmissible diseases.

From the passage, "Infectious pathologies are also called communicable diseases or transmissible diseases, due to their potential of transmission from one person or species to another by a replicating agent (as opposed to a toxin)."

3. C
Infectivity describes the ability of an organism to enter, survive and multiply in the host. This is taken directly from the passage, and is a definition type question.

Definition type questions can be answered quickly and easily by scanning the passage for the word you are asked to define.

"Infectivity" is an unusual word, so it is quick and easy to scan the passage looking for this word.

4. B
We know an infection is not synonymous with an infectious disease because an infection may not cause important clinical symptoms or impair host function.

5. C
We can infer from the passage that, a virus is too small to be seen with the naked eye. Clearly, if they are too small

to be seen with a microscope, then they are too small to be seen with the naked eye.

6. D

Viruses infect all types of organisms. This is taken directly from the passage, "Viruses infect all types of organisms, from animals and plants to bacteria and single-celled organisms."

7. C

The passage does not say exactly how many parts prions and viroids consist of. It does say, "Unlike prions and viroids, viruses consist of two or three parts ..." so we can infer they consist of either less than two or more than three parts.

8. B

A common virus spread by coughing and sneezing is Influenza.

9. C

The cumulus stage of a thunderstorm is the beginning of the thunderstorm.

This is taken directly from the passage, "The first stage of a thunderstorm is the cumulus, or developing stage."

10. D

The passage lists four ways that air is heated. One ways is heat created by water vapor condensing into liquid.

11. A

The sequence of events can be taken from these sentences:

As the moisture carried by the [1] air currents rises, it rapidly cools into liquid drops of water, which appear as cumulus clouds. As the water vapor condenses into liquid, it [2] releases heat, which warms the air. This in turn causes the air to become less dense than the surrounding dry air and [3] rise further.

12. C

The purpose of this text is to explain when meteorologists consider a thunderstorm severe.

The main idea is the first sentence, "The United States National Weather Service classifies thunderstorms as severe when they reach a predetermined level." After the first sentence, the passage explains and elaborates on this idea. Everything is this passage is related to this idea, and there are no other major ideas in this passage that are central to the whole passage.

13. A
From this passage, we can infer that different areas and countries have different criteria for determining a severe storm.

From the passage we can see that most of the US has a criteria of, winds over 50 knots (58 mph or 93 km/h), and hail ¾ inch (2 cm). For the Central US, hail must be 1 inch (2.5 cm) in diameter. In Canada, winds must be 90 km/h or greater, hail 2 centimeters in diameter or greater, and rainfall more than 50 millimeters in 1 hour, or 75 millimeters in 3 hours.

Option D is incorrect because the Canadian system is the same for hail, 2 centimeters in diameter.

14. C
With hail above the minimum size of 2.5 cm. diameter, the Central Region of the United States National Weather Service would issue a severe thunderstorm warning.

15. D
Clouds in space are made of different materials attracted by gravity. Clouds on Earth are made of water droplets or ice crystals.

Choice D is the best answer. Notice also that Choice D is the most specific.

16. C
The main idea is the first sentence of the passage; a cloud is a visible mass of droplets or frozen crystals floating in the atmosphere above the surface of the Earth or other planetary body.

The main idea is very often the first sentence of the paragraph.

17. C
Nephology, which is the study of cloud physics.

18. C
This question asks about the process, and gives options that can be confirmed or eliminated easily.

From the passage, "Dense, deep clouds reflect most light, so they appear white, at least from the top. Cloud droplets scatter light very efficiently, so the farther into a cloud light travels, the weaker it gets. This accounts for the gray or dark appearance at the base of large clouds."

We can eliminate choice A, since water droplets inside the cloud do not reflect light is false.

We can eliminate choice B, since, water droplets outside the cloud reflect light, it appears dark, is false.

Choice C is correct.

19. A
Low blood sugar occurs both in diabetics and healthy adults.

20. B
None of the statements are the author's opinion.

21. A
The author's purpose is to inform.

22. A
The only statement that is not a detail is, "A doctor can diagnosis this medical condition by asking the patient questions and testing."

23. B
The general tone is informal.

24. B
The statement, " Fewer people have aquariums in their office than at home," cannot be inferred from this article.

25. C
The author does not provide evidence for this statement.

26. A
Navy SEALS are the maritime component of the United States Special Operations Command (USSOCOM).

27. C
Working underwater separates SEALs from other military units. This is taken directly from the passage.

28. D
SEALs also belong to the Navy and the Coast Guard.

29. A
The CIA also participated. From the passage, the raid was conducted by a "team of 40 *CIA-led* Navy SEALS."

30. C
From the passage, "The Navy SEALs were part of the Naval Special Warfare Development Group, previously called 'Team 6.' "

31. B
This question is taken directly from the passage.

32. A
The Egyptians believed gods loved gardens.

33. B
Cypresses and palms were the most popular trees in Assyrian Gardens.
34. B
Vegetable gardens came before ornamental gardens.

The earliest forms of gardens emerged from the people's need to grow herbs and vegetables. It was only later that rich individuals created gardens for the purely decorative purpose.

35. A
Secede most nearly means to break away from because the 11 states wanted to leave the United States and form their own country.

D is incorrect because the states seceded before they lost

the war.

36. B
Look at the dates in the passage. The shots were fired on
April 12 and Congress declared war on April 14.

Option A is incorrect because the dates show clearly which
happened first. Option
C is incorrect because the passage states that Lincoln was
against slavery. Option
D is incorrect because it never mentions who was or was
not at Fort Sumter.

37. C
The passage clearly states that Lee surrendered to Grant
after the capture of the capital of the Confederacy, which is
Richmond.

Option A is incorrect because the war continued for 2 years
after Gettysburg. Option B is incorrect because that battle
is not mentioned in the passage. Option D is incorrect
because the capture of the capital occurred after the march
to the sea.

38. A
When the passage said that the North had abolished slavery, it implies that slaves were no longer allowed to be had
in the North. In essence slavery was banned.

39. C
To be infamous means to be remembered for an evil or terrible action. Therefore, the word infamy means to remember a bad or terrible thing.

Option A is incorrect because being famous is not the same
as being infamous

40. C
Each other answer set contains the name of at least one
country who was not part of the AXIS powers.

41. D
The correct option is stated in the passage.

42. C
The passage clearly states that Japan planned a surprise attack. They chose that early time to catch the U.S. military off guard.

43. B
The correct answer can be found in the fourth sentence of the first paragraph.

Option A is incorrect because repenting begins the day AFTER Mardi Gras.
Option C is incorrect because you can celebrate Mardi Gras without being a member of a Krewe.

44. A
The second sentence is the last paragraph states that Krewes are led by the Kings and Queens. Therefore, you must have to be part of a Krewe to be its King or its Queen.

Option B is incorrect because it never states in the passage that only people from France can be Kings and Queen of Mardi Gras. Option C is incorrect because the passage says nothing about having to speak French.

45. C
The first sentences of BOTH the 2nd and 3rd paragraphs mention that French explorers started this tradition in New Orleans.

Options A, B and D are incorrect because they are just names of cities or countries listed in the 2nd paragraph.

Section II – Mathematics

1. A
1/3 X 3/4 = 3/12 = 1/4

2. D
75/1500 = 15/300 = 3/60 = 1/20

3. D
3.14 + 2.73 = 5.87 and 5.87 + 23.7 = 29.57

4. B
Spent 15% - 100% - 15% = 85%

5. C
To convert a decimal to a fraction, take the places of decimal as your denominator, in this case 2, so in 0.27, '7' is in the 100th place, so the fraction is 27/100 and 0.33 becomes 33/100.

Next estimate the answer quickly to eliminate obvious wrong choices. 27/100 is about 1/4 and 33/100 is 1/3. 1/3 is slightly larger than 1/4, and 1/4 + 1/4 is 1/2, so the answer will be slightly larger than 1/2.

Looking at the choices, Choice A can be eliminated since 3/6 = 1/2. Choice D, 2/7 is less than 1/2 and can also be eliminated. So the answer is going to be Choice B or Choice C.

Do the calculation, 0.27 + 0.33 = 0.60 and 0.60 = 60/100 = 3/5, Choice C is correct.

6. D
3.13 + 7.87 = 11 and 11 X 5 = 55

7. B
2/4 X 3/4 = 6/16, and lowest terms = 3/8

8. D
2/3 - 2/5 = 10 - 6/15 = 4/15

9. C
2/7 + 2/3 = 6+14 /21 (21 is the common denominator) = 20/21

10. B
2/3 x 60 = 40 and 1.5 x 75 = 15, 40 + 15 = 55

11. C
This is an easy question, and shows how you can solve some questions without doing the calculations. The question is, 8 is what percent of 40. Take easy percentages for an approximate answer and see what you get.

10% is easy to calculate because you can drop the zero, or move the decimal point.   10% of 40 = 4, and 8 = 2 X 4, so, 8 must be 2 X 10% = 20%.

Here are the calculations which confirm the quick approximation.
8/40 = X/100 = 8 * 100 / 40X = 800/40 = X = 20

12. D
This is the same type of question which illustrates another method to solve quickly without doing the calculations. The question is, 9 is what percent of 36?

Ask, what is the relationship between 9 and 36? 9 X 4 = 36 so they are related by a factor of 4. If 9 is related to 36 by a factor of 4, then what is related to 100 (to get a percent) by a factor of 4?

To visualize:

9 X 4 = 36
Z X 4 = 100

So the answer is 25. 9 has the same relation to 36 as 25 has to 100.

Here are the calculations which confirm the quick approximation.
9/36 = X/100 = 9 * 100 / 36X = 900/36 = 25%.

13. C
3/10 * 90 = 3 * 90/10 = 27

14. B
.4/100 * 36 = .4 * 36/100 = .144

15. A
5 mg/10/mg X 1 tab/1 = .5 tablets

16. B
Step 1: Set up the formula to calculate the dose to be given in mg as per weight of the child:-
Dose ordered X Weight in Kg = Dose to be given
Step 2: 20 mg X 12 kg = 240 mg

240 mg/80 mg X 1 tab/1 = 240/80 = 3 tablets

17. A
Set up the formula to calculate the dose to be given in mg as per weight of the child:-
Dose ordered X Weight in Kg = Dose to be given
Step 2: 20 mg X 20 kg = 400 mg (Convert 44 lb to Kg, 1 lb = 0.4536 kg, hence 44 lb = 19.95 kg approx. 20 kg)
400 mg/80 mg X 1 tab/1 = 400/80 = 5 tablets

18. B
3000 units/5000 units X 1 ml/1 = 3000/5000 = 0.6 ml

19. C
60 mg/80 mg X 1 ml/1 = 60/80 = 0.75 ml

20. A
Dose ordered X Weight in Kg = Dose to be given
16 mg X 15 kg = 240 mg
240 mg/80 mg X 1 tab/1 = 240/80 = 3 tablets

21. C
(Convert 1 g = 1000 mg)
1000 mg/1000 mg X 1 tsp/1 = 1000/1000 = 1 tsp

22. D
10 units/200 units X 1 ml/1 = 10/200 = 0.05 ml

23. B
$(4)(3)^3 = (4)(27) = 108$

24. A
1000g = 1kg., 0.007 = 1000 x 0.007 = 7g.

25. C
4 quarts = 1 gallon, 16 quarts = 16/4 = 4 gallons

26. C
1 teaspoon = 4.93 milliliters (U.S.), 2 tp = 4.93 x 2 = 9.86 ml.

27. D
1,000 meters = 1 kilometer, 200 m = 200/1,000 = 0.2 km.

28. B
12 inches = 1 ft., 72 inches = 72/12 = 6 feet

29. C
1 yard = 3 feet, 3 yards = 3 feet x 3 = 9 feet

30. B
0.45 kg = 1 pound, 1 kg. = 1/0.45 and 45 kg = 1/0.45 x 45
= 45 = 100 pounds.

31. C
1 g = 1,000 mg. 0.63 g = 0.63 x 1,000 = 630 mg.

32. D
To solve for x,
5x – 7x + 3 = -1
5x – 7x = -1 -3
-2x = -4
x = -4/ -2
x = 2

33. C
To solve for x, first simplify the equation
5x + 2x + 14 = 14x – 7
7x + 14 = 4x -7
7x – 14x + 14 = -7
7x – 14x = -7 – 14
-7x = -21
x = -21/-7
x=3

34. A
5z + 5 = 3z +6 + 11
5z -3z + 5 =6 + 11
5z – 3z = 6 + 11 -5
2z = 17 – 5
2z = 12
z= 12/2
z= 6

35. C
5z + 5 = 3z +6 + 11
5z -3z + 5 =6 + 11
5z – 3z = 6 + 11 -5

$2z = 17 - 5$
$2z = 12$
$z = 12/2$
$z = 6$

36. D
Price increased by \$5 (\$25-\$20). The percent increase is $5/20$ x $100 = 500/20 = 25\%$.

37. C
Price decreased by \$5 (\$25-\$20). The percent decrease = $5/25$ x $100 = 5$ x $4 = 20\%$.

38. D
$30/100$ x $150 = 3$ x $15 = 45$ (increase in number of correct answers). So the number of correct answers in second test $= 150 + 45 = 195$

39. B
Let total number of players = X
Let the number of players with long hair=Y and the number of players with short hair=Z
Then $X = 4 + Z$
$Y = 12\%$ of X
$Z = X - 4$
12.5% of $X = 4$
Converting from decimal to fraction gives $12.5\% = 125/10$ x $1/100 = 125/1000$, therefore 12.5% of $= 125/1000X = 4$
Solve for X by multiplying both sides by $1000/125$, $X = 4$ x $1000/125 = 32$
$Z = x - 4$
$Z = 32 - 4$
z or number of short haired players = 28

40. D
2 glasses are broken for 43 customers so 1 glass breaks for every $43/2$ customers served, therefore 10 glasses implies $(43/2) \cdot 10 = 215$ customers.

41. D
As the lawn is square , the length of one side will be the square root of the area. $\sqrt{62,500} = 250$ meters. So, the perimeter is found by 4 times the length of the side of the square:

250•4 = 1000 meters.

Since each meter costs \$5.5, the total cost of the fence will be 1000•5.5 = \$5,500.

42. D
The price of all the single items is same and there are 13 total items. So the total cost will be 13 × 1.3 = \$16.9. After 3.5 percent tax this amount will become 16.9 × 1.035 = \$17.5.

43. C
Area of the square = 12 × 12 = 144 cm²
Let x be the width, then 2x be the length of rectangle, so its area will be $2x^2$ and perimeter will be 2(2x + x) = 6x
According to the condition
$2x^2$ = 144
X = 8.48 cm
The perimeter will be
Perimeter = 6 × 8.48
= 50.88
= 51 cm.

44. B
There are 50 balls in the basket now. Let x be the number of yellow balls to be added to make 65%. So the equation becomes

X + 15 /X + 50 = 65/100
X = 50

45. D
Let x be number of rows, and number of trees in a row. So equation becomes
X^2 = 65536
X = 256

46. A
The distribution is done in three different rates and amounts:

\$6.4 per 20 kilograms to 15 shops ... 20•15 = 300 kilograms distributed

\$3.4 per 10 kilograms to 12 shops ... 10•12 = 120

kilograms distributed

550 - (300 + 120) = 550 - 420 = 130 kilograms left. This amount is distributed by 5 kilogram portions. So, this means that there are 130/5 = 26 shops.

$1.8 per 130 kilograms.

We need to find the amount he earned overall these distributions.

$6.4 per 20 kilograms : 6.4•15 = $96 for 300 kilograms

$3.4 per 10 kilograms : 3.4•12 = $40.8 for 120 kilograms

$1.8 per 5 kilograms : 1.8•26 = $46.8 for 130 kilograms

So, he earned 96 + 40.8 + 46.8 = $ 183.6

The total distribution cost is given as $10

The profit is found by: Money earned - money spent ... It is important to remember that he bought 550 kilograms of potatoes for $165 at the beginning:

Profit = 183.6 - 10 - 165 = $8.6

47. D
Each tree will require a 10-meter diametric space around its stem. So 65 trees can be planted along 650-meter side. Similarly, 65 along the other side. However, along the 780 meter side, the first tree will be after 10 meters at both edges, so 76 trees can be planted long that side.

Total number of trees then will be 65×2+76×2=282

48. D
1 foot is equal to 12 inches. So 1 ft^2 = 12•12 in^2

4 ft^2 = 4•12•12 in^2 = 576 in^2

This amount of surface area is divided equally among 3 boys.

Each boy will clean 576/3 = 192 in^2

192 in^2 = 144 in^2 + 48 in^2; 144 in^2 = 1 ft^2

So, each boy will clean 1 ft^2 and 48 in^2

49. B

We check the fractions taking place in the question. We see that there is a "half" (that is $1/2$) and $3/7$. So, we multiply the denominators of these fractions to decide how to name the total money. We say that Mr. Johnson has 14x at the beginning; he gives half of this, meaning 7x, to his family. $250 to his landlord. He has $3/7$ of his money left. $3/7$ of 14x is equal to:

$14x \cdot (3/7) = 6x$

So,

Spent money is: $7x + 250$

Unspent money is: $6x$

Total money is: $14x$

We write an equation: total money = spent money + unspent money

$14x = 7x + 250 + 6x$

$14x - 7x - 6x = 250$

$x = 250$

We are asked to find the total money that is 14x:

$14x = 14 \cdot 250 = \$3500$

50. A

The probability that the 1st ball drawn is red $= 4/11$
The probability that the 2nd ball drawn is green $= 5/10$
The combined probability will then be $4/11 \times 5/10 = 20/110 = 2/11$

Section III English Grammar

1. A
The third conditional is used for talking about an unreal situation (a situation that did not happen) in the past. For example, "If I had studied harder, [if clause] I would have passed the exam" [main clause]. This has the same meaning as, "I failed the exam, because I didn't study hard enough."

2. A
A Pronoun should conform to its antecedent in gender, number and person.

3. C
The verb might is used to express possibility or permission when in the past tense. May is the present tense of might.

4. C
In double negative sentences, one of the negatives is replaced with "any."

5. C
Words such as neither, each, many, either, every, everyone, everybody and any should take a singular pronoun.

6. C
The present perfect tense cannot be used with specific time expressions such as yesterday, one year ago, last week, when I was a child, at that moment, that day, one day, etc. The present perfect tense is used with unspecific expressions such as ever, never, once, many times, several times, before, so far, already, yet, etc.

7. A
"Went" is used in the simple past tense. "Gone" is used in the past perfect tense.

8. C
Although 'can' can be used to mean the same thing as 'may,' the difference is that 'can' is used for negative or interrogative sentences, while 'may' is used in affirmative

sentences to express possibility.

9. C
Words such as neither, each, many, either, every, everyone, everybody and any should take a singular pronoun. Here we are assuming that the subject is female, and so use "her." The subject could be male, in which case we would use "his," however that is not a choice here.

10. C
"It's" is a contraction for it is or it has. "Its" is a possessive pronoun.

11. B
The sentence refers to a person, so "who" is the only correct option.

12. A
The sentence requires the past perfect "has always been known." Furthermore, this is the only grammatically correct choice.

13. B
"Will" is used in the second or third person (they, he, she and you), while "shall" is used in the first person (I and we). Both verbs are used to express futurity. In common usage and everyday conversation, however, they can be interchanged.

14. D
When comparing two items, use "the taller." When comparing more than two items, use "the tallest."

15. B
The past perfect form is used to describe an event that occurred in the past and prior to another event. Here there are two things that happened, both of them in the past, and something the person wanted to do.

Event 1: Kiss came to town
Event 2: All the tickets sold out
What I wanted to do: Buy a ticket

The events are arranged:

When KISS came to town, all of the tickets had been sold out before I could buy one.

16. A
The subject is "rules" so the present tense plural form, "are," is used to agree with "realize."

17. A
Use "whom" in the objective case, and use "who" a subjective case.

18. D
The simple past tense, "sank," is correct because it refers to completed action in the past.

19. A
"Who" is correct because the question uses an active construction. "To whom was first place given?" is passive construction.

20. D
"Which" is correct, because the files are objects and not people.

21. C
The simple present tense, "rises," is correct.

22. A
"Lie" does not require a direct object, while "lay" does. The old woman might lie on the couch, which has no direct object, or she might lay the book down, which has the direct object, "the book."

23. D
The simple present tense, "falls," is correct because it is repeated action.

24. A
The present progressive, "building models," is correct in this sentence; it is required to match the other present progressive verbs.

25. A
"Affect" is a verb, while "effect" is a noun.

26. D
"Than" is used for comparison. "Then" is used to indicate a point in time.

27. C
"There" indicates a state of existence. "Their" is used for third person plural possession. "They're" is the contracted form of "they are."

28. A
The verb "ought" can be used to express desirability, duty and probability. The verb is usually followed by "to."

29. A
When you use 'each other' it should be used for two things or people. When you use 'one another' it should be used for more than two things or people.

30. C
"Your" is the possessive form of "you." "You're" is the contraction of "you are."

31. A
Disease is a singular noun.

32. C
Both "dog" and "cat" in this sentence are singular nouns and require the article "a."

33. A
The word "principal" is a synonym for primary or major. "Principle" means a fundamental truth.

34. D
The article "a" come before a noun that begins with a consonant, while "an" comes before a noun that begins with a vowel.

35. A
"Except" means to exclude something. "Accept" means to receive something, or to agree to an idea.

36. A
"Advise" is a verb that means to offer advice, which is a noun.

37. C
"Adapt" means to change or accommodate. "Adopt" means to accept, embrace, or to assume responsibility or ownership for something or someone.

38. D
"Among" is used with more than two items, while "between" is limited to two items.

39. D
"At" refers to a specific time or location, while "about" is approximate.

40. B
"Beside" means next to, and "besides" means in addition to.

41. A
"Can" is used when describing ability or capability. "May" is a request or the granting of permission.

42. B
"Continuous" means a time period without interruption, or ongoing. "Continual" is used for actions that are frequent and repetitive, or that continue almost without interruption.

43. A
"Emigrate" means to leave one's country, usually to immigrate to another country to live.

44. A
"Farther" is reserved for physical distance, and "further" is used for figurative distance, or to mean "in addition."

45. B
"Former" refers to the first of two things; "latter" to the second of two things.

46. D
"Healthy" describes people or animals that are in good health. "Healthful" is generally used in formal speech or writing, and refers to things that are good for health.

47. C
"Lie" does not require a direct object, while "lay" does. In this sentence, "lay" is followed by the direct object, "the books."

48. C
"Lie" does not require a direct object, while "lay" does. In this sentence, "lay" is followed by the direct object, "the books."

49. C
This is the correct choice.

50. A
"Learn" means to receive and integrate knowledge or an experience. "Teach" means to impart knowledge to another.

Section IV Vocabulary

1. C
Dauntless: adj. Invulnerable to fear or intimidation.

2. A
Juxtaposed: adj. Placed side-by-side often for comparison or contrast.

3. B
Regicide: v. killing of a king.

4. A
Pernicious: adj. Causing much harm in a subtle way.

5. A
Immune: adj. Resistant to a particular infection or toxin owing to the presence of specific antibodies.

6. B
Nimble: adj. Quick and light in movement or action.

7. A
Queries: n. Questions or inquiries.

8. C
Depose: To remove (a leader) from (high) office, without killing the incumbent.

9. D
Pedestrian: Ordinary, dull; everyday; unexceptional.

10. B
Petulant: adj. Childishly irritable.

11. D
Pesticide: n. A substance used for destroying insects or other organisms harmful to cultivated plants or to animals.

12. D
Salient: adj. worthy or note or relevant.

13. B
Sedentary: adj. not moving or sitting in one place.

14. A
Famine: n. extreme scarcity of food.

15. A
Stint: n. To be sparing.

16. A
Precipitate: v. to rain.

17. C
Edify: v. To instruct or improve morally or intellectually.

18. B
Egress: n. An exit or way out.

19. A
Recede: v. To move back, to move away.

20. A
Confidential: adj. kept secret within a certain circle of persons; not intended to be known publicly.

21. A
Aggravate: v. to make worse, or more severe; to render less tolerable or less excusable; to make more offensive; to enhance; to intensify.

22. B
Debut: n. a performer's first-time performance to the public.

23. B
Hormones: n. A regulatory substance produced in an

organism and transported in tissue fluids such as blood or sap to stimulate specific cells.

24. B
Importune: v. To harass with persistent requests.

25. B
Sedulous: adj. Showing dedication and diligence.

26. A
Tincture: n. alcoholic drink with plant extracts used for medicine.

27. C
Felony: n. Serious criminal offence that is punishable by death or imprisonment above a year.

28. A
Bibliophile: n. One who loves books.

29. A
Monsoons: n. The rainy season accompanying the wet monsoon.

30. D
Volatile: adj. Explosive.

31. B
Plaintive: adj. Sorrowful, mournful or melancholic.

32. B
Truism: n. Self evident or clear obvious truth.

33. B
Foment: v. to encourage or incite troublesome acts.

34. A
Funereal: Adj. dignified, solemn that is appropriate for a funeral.

35. A
Flagrant: obvious and offensive, blatant, scandalous.

36. B
Moss

37. A
Nexus: n. A connection or series of connections linking two or more things.

38. A
Zealot: n. A person who is very passionate and fanatic about his specific objectives or beliefs.

39. B
Vertigo: n. Dizziness.

40. A
Trenchant: adj. Vigorous or incisive in expression or style.

41. B
Geniality: n. warmth and kindness of disposition.

42. A
Habitual: adj. Behaving in a regular manner, as a habit.

43. B
Idolize: v. To make an idol of, or to worship as an idol.

44. C
Osculate: v. to kiss or related to kissing.

45. D
Conjoin: v. To join; to unite; to combine.

46. B
Petrify: v. To harden organic matter by permeating with water and depositing dissolved minerals.

47. A
Extinguish: v. Cause a fire or light to cease to burn or shine.

48. C
Convection: n. Heat transfer in a gas or liquid by the circulation of currents.

49. A
Intrepid: adj. Fearless; adventurous.

50. D
Goad: v. To encourage, stimulate or incite and provoke.

Section V – Science

1. A
The formula for acceleration = A = $(V_f - V_0)/t$
so A = $(120 - 90)/5$ sec = 5 mph/second^2

2. A
Only genetics pertains directly to the cell's function. For genetics, the cell of a new organism acquires traits of ancestral organisms.

3. A
A solution with a pH value of greater than 7 is base.

4. B
The voltage across a resistor is equal to the product of the resistance and the current flowing through it.

5. A
Eukaryotic and prokaryotic cells are both organelles.

6. C
Electric potential is a fundamental interaction between the magnetic field and the presence and motion of an electric charge.

Electric potential is the capacity of an electric field to do work on an electric charge, typically measured in volts, while electromagnetism is a fundamental interaction between the magnetic field and the presence and motion of an electric charge.

7. C
Subversion. Active transport, adhesion and cell signaling are all involved in cellular biology.

8. C
Homologous is being inherited by the organisms' common ancestors. An example would be feathers and hair—both of which were structures that shared a common ancestral trait.

9. C
The manner in which instructions for building proteins, the basic structural molecules of living material are written in the DNA is a **genetic code**.

10. C
A gene is a unit of inherited material, encoded by a strand of DNA and transcribed by RNA.

11. B
Speed = (total distance traveled)/(total time taken)
6 = x/120   (convert minutes to seconds)
6 * 120 = x
X = 720 meters

12. D

Cellular scientists' biographies are not studied in cell biology. The physiological properties of cells, cell structure and the life cycle of a cell are all valid topics of study within the field of cell biology.

13. A

Detection of pathogens can be complicated because they evolve so quickly.

14. C

Molarity = moles of solute/liters of solution = 8/4 = 2

15. D

An ohm (Ω) is a unit of electrical voltage is not true.

Note: An ohm is a unit of electrical resistance.

16. D

The periodic table as it is now contains 118 elements.

17. C

Mutations in DNA sequences usually occur spontaneously is false.

Note: Mutations result when the DNA polymerase makes a mistake, which happens about once every 100,000,000 bases. Actually, the number of mistakes that remain incorporated into the DNA is even lower than this because cells contain special DNA repair proteins that fix many of the mistakes in the DNA that are caused by mutagens. The repair proteins see which nucleotides are paired incorrectly, and then change the wrong base to the right one. [7]

18. C

Momentum is a product of velocity and mass. If they are all traveling at the same speed, the car that weighs the most would have the highest momentum.

19. A

Starting with the weakest, the fundamental forces of nature in order of strength are, Gravity, Weak nuclear force, Electromagnetic force, Strong nuclear force.

Note: Although gravitational force is the weakest of the four, it acts over great distances. Electromagnetic force is of order 10^{39} times stronger than gravity.

20. A
Electrons are subatomic particles that carry a negative charge.

21. A
Cell culture is the technique for growing cells independent of a living organism within the confines of a laboratory. The cell culture is generally grown in a test-tube environment or on a petri dish.

22. A
Precision, which refers to the repeatability of measurement, does not require knowledge of the correct or true value.

23. C
All conductors contain electrical charges, which will move when an electric potential difference (measured in volts) is applied across separate points on the material. This flow of charge (measured in amperes) is what is meant by electric current.

24. B
The periodic table is a tabular display of the chemical elements, organized on the basis of their atomic numbers, electron configurations, and recurring chemical properties.

25. D
The scientific discipline that studies the physiological aspects, structures, life cycles and division of cells is called cell biology.

26. A
Ionization energy is the minimum amount of energy required to remove an electron from an atom or ion in the gas phase.

27. C
Redox is a complete reaction comprising oxidation and reduction reactions that are each only half of the complete reaction. The same exact electrons lost in oxidation are what are gained in reduction.

28. A
In terms of the scientific method, the term **observation** refers to the act of noticing or perceiving something and/or recording a fact or occurrence.

29. B
The Lewis Theory defines acids and bases in terms of the electron-pair concept; according to its definition, an acid is an electron-pair acceptor, and a base is an electron-pair donor.

30. A
First convert 250 ml to liters, 250/1000 = 0.25 then calculate molarity = 5 moles/ 0.25 liters = 20 M.

31. D
The property of a conductor that restricts its internal flow of electrons is resistance.

32. A
Prokaryotic microorganisms that are usually just a few micrometers long.

33. B
Kinetic energy is the energy of a body that results from motion while potential energy is the energy possessed by an object by virtue of its position or state, e.g., as in a compressed spring.

34. B
The formula for acceleration = $A = (V_f - V_0)/t$
so A = (2000 - 0)/25 sec = 80 m/sec^2

35. D
The four states in which matter exists are solid, liquid, gas, and plasma.

The state of matter is determined by the strength of the bonds between the atoms that make up matter.

36. A
The cell membrane is a biological membrane that separates the interior of all cells from the outside environment. The cell membrane is selectively permeable to ions and organic molecules and controls the movement of substances in and out of cells. [8]

37. C
Electric current is the flow of electric charge through a medium.

38. D
Cubes rarely occur naturally, especially in the micro world outside of the human eye. True cubes are usually deliberately created.

39. D
All acids contain hydrogen. When acids react with most metals, the metals displace the hydrogen and hydrogen gas is produced.

40. D
Relative position. Ranks include Domain, Kingdom, Phylum, Class, Order, Family, Genus, and Species.

41. B
The following statements about the periodic table of the elements is true,
The way in which the elements are arranged allows for predictions to made about their behavior.

42. D
The scientific term **experiment** refers to a practical test designed with the intention that its results be relevant to a particular theory or set of theories.

43. B
Substances that deactivate catalysts are called catalytic poisons.

44. B
Atmospheric pressure is the force per unit area exerted against a surface by the weight of air above that surface in the Earth's atmosphere.

45. B
Kinetic energy is the energy an object possesses due to its motion.

46. D
Scientific classification. The two phrases are interchangeable, although the former seems to more accurately reflect the purpose of classification: to categorize biological units.

47. D
Oxidation and reduction reactions are each just half of a redox reaction and both occur simultaneously, because

the exact electrons lost in oxidation is what is gained in reduction.

48. C

A recessive gene is not expressed as a trait unless inherited by both parents.

49. D

A **scientific model** is an approximation or simulation of a real system that omits all but the most essential variables of the system.

50. A

A positively charged subatomic particle forming part of the nucleus of an atom and determining the atomic number of an element.

51. A

Neutrons are necessary within an atomic nucleus as they bind with protons via the nuclear force.

52. A

Atoms of different elements combine in simple whole-number ratios to form chemical compounds.

53. C

The following statement is false - Most enzymes are inorganic.

54. C

Acids are compounds that contain hydrogen and can dissolve in water to release hydrogen ions into solution.

55. B

Formula - P= kg x m/s
= 12.05kg x 8m/s
= 96.4 kg x m/s down the hill.

Note that the final answer has the proper SI unit of momentum (kg x m/s) after it and it also mentions the direction of the movement.

56. D

All of the statements are true.

> a. A non-metal is a substance that conducts heat and electricity poorly.

b. The majority of the known chemical elements are non-metals.

c. A non-metal is brittle or waxy or gaseous.

57. B
The discipline that studies bacteria is Bacteriology.

58. A
Genes determine individual hereditary characteristics.

59. C
A and B are true.

a. Light consists of electromagnetic waves in the visible range.

b. The fundamental particle or quantum of light is a photon.

Note: Light energy is the only visible form of energy. A light bulb is a device that uses electrical energy to create electromagnetic energy in the form (in part) of visible light and heat.

60. A
The groups into which organisms are classified are called taxa and include, in order of size, Genus, Kingdom, Phylum/division, Class, Order, and Family Species.

61. A
Chemical bonds are attractions between atoms that form chemical substances containing two or more atoms.

62. C
In chemistry, the number of protons in the nucleus of an atom is known as the atomic number, which determines the chemical element to which the atom belongs.

63. D
The molarity of an aqueous solution of CaCl is defined as the moles of CaCl per liter of solution.

64. C
An electron is a tiny particle with a negative charge that orbits a nucleus.

65. C
The Law of the Conservation of Energy states that, in a chemical change, energy can be neither created nor destroyed, but only changed from one form to another.

66. A

An atom is the basic or fundamental unit of any matter or element.

67. A

Females have two X chromosomes and males have one X chromosome and one Y chromosome.

68. A

A biofilm is a dense aggregation of bacteria attached to surfaces. The density of these bacteria is based on many factors, such as environment, temperature, and how long they're left there undisturbed.

69. A

Water has two hydrogen atoms covalently bonded to one oxygen atom.

70. A

Electrical resistance is measured in Ohms.

71. A

First convert LiF grams to moles = 52 x 1/26 = 2. Now Molarity = 2 moles/2.5 liters = 0.8 M

72. C

In physics, friction is the force that opposes the relative motion of two bodies in contact.

73. D

Anabolism is the series of chemical reactions resulting in the synthesis of organic compounds, and catabolism is a series of chemical reactions that break down larger molecules.

74. C

When an acid and a base react, they neutralize each other's properties to form salt and water.

75. A

Reduction is a reaction that usually involves the gain of electrons that were lost in an oxidation reaction.

Section VI - Anatomy and Physiology

1. A
The Left upper quadrant of the abdomen, is often abbreviated as LUQ, contains the stomach, spleen, left lobe of the liver, body of the pancreas, left kidney and adrenal gland.

2. A
Human homeostasis is the ability of the body to regulate its **inner environment** in response to fluctuations in the environment outside the body.

3. B
Epithelial tissue acts as a **protective barrier for the human body**.

4. C
The integumentary system is the organ system that protects the body from damage, comprising the skin and its appendages, including hair, scales, feathers, and nails.

5. D
Another primary purpose of the musculoskeletal system is **providing form for the body**.

6. B
The circulatory system is an organ system that passes nutrients (such as amino acids, electrolytes and lymph), gases, hormones, blood cells, etc. to and from cells in the body to help fight diseases and help stabilize body temperature and pH to maintain homeostasis.

7. B
The lungs are an important component of the respiratory system.

8. A
The immune system fight off disease by identifying and killing tumor cells and pathogens.

9. D
The primary purpose of the digestive system is to convert food into a form that can provide nourishment for the body.

10. B
Urine is mostly comprised of waste material after the body has taken the nutrients from food and absorbed the water

it needs.

11. A
The gallbladder is located in the Right Upper Quadrant together with the liver, right kidney, colon, pancreas and large intestine.

12. A
The lymphatic system is defined as the system which carries a clear liquid lymph toward the heart.

13. A
The spleen is an organ found in virtually all vertebrate animals with important roles in regard to red blood cells (also referred to as erythrocytes) and the immune system. In humans it is located in the left upper quadrant of the abdomen. It removes old red blood cells and holds a reserve of blood in case of hemorrhagic shock while also recycling iron.[9]

14. D
The right upper quadrant of the abdomen, often abbreviated as RUQ, contains the liver, gall bladder, duodenum and had of the pancreas.

15. B
Exercise and low fat diets will increase metabolism. Choice B, **a man who is past 30 and whose body is losing muscle** is the only choice.

16. C
Muscle tissue has the ability to **relax and contract**, bringing out movement and the ability to work.

17. C
The human skin (integumentary) is composed of a minimum of 3 major layers of tissue, the Epidermis, the Dermis and Hypodermis.

18. A
Cartilage is a flexible connective tissue found in many areas in the bodies of humans and other animals, including the joints between bones, the rib cage, the ear, the nose, the elbow, the knee, the ankle, the bronchial tubes and the intervertebral discs. It is not as hard and rigid as bone but is stiffer and less flexible than muscle. [10]

19. A
The main components of the circulatory system are the

heart, veins and blood vessels.

20. D
The exchange of oxygen for carbon dioxide takes place in the alveolar area of the lungs.

21. A
Detection of pathogens can be complicated because **they evolve so quickly**.

22. B
Cleansing food of impurities is not an example of a function of the stomach in digestion.

23. A
Urea is the name of the waste removed from the body through urine.

24. C
An example of an organ that plays a big role in the lymphatic system is the spleen.

25. C
The central nervous system (CNS) is the part of the nervous system that integrates the information that it receives from and coordinates the activity of all parts of the bodies of bi-laterian animals—that is all multi-cellular animals except sponges and radially symmetric animals such as jellyfish. It contains the majority of the nervous system and consists of the brain and the spinal cord. Some classifications also include the retina and the cranial nerves in the CNS. Together with the peripheral nervous system it has a fundamental role in the control of behavior. [11]

Practice Test Questions Set 2

Section I – Reading Comprehension

Questions: 45
Time: 60 Minutes

Section II – Mathematics

Questions: 50
Time: 60 Minutes

Section III English Grammar

Questions: 50
Time: 50 Minutes

Section IV - Vocabulary

Questions: 50
Time: 50 Minutes

Section V – Part I – Science

Questions: 75
Time: 125 minutes

Section VI Anatomy & Physiology

Questions: 25
Time: 25 minutes

The practice test portion presents questions that are representative of the type of question you should expect to find on the HESI®. However, they are not intended to match exactly what is on the HESI®.

For the best results, take this Practice Test as if it were the real exam. Set aside time when you will not be disturbed, and a location that is quiet and free of distractions. Read the instructions carefully, read each question carefully, and answer to the best of your ability.

Use the bubble answer sheets provided. When you have completed the Practice Test, check your answer against the Answer Key and read the explanation provided.

Do not attempt more than one set of practice test questions in one day. After completing the first practice test, wait two or three days before attempting the second set of questions.

This set of practice test questions contains ALL of the HESI® modules. Different schools use different modules so be sure to check with your school for the modules being used.

Reading Comprehension

1. (A) (B) (C) (D)
2. (A) (B) (C) (D)
3. (A) (B) (C) (D)
4. (A) (B) (C) (D)
5. (A) (B) (C) (D)
6. (A) (B) (C) (D)
7. (A) (B) (C) (D)
8. (A) (B) (C) (D)
9. (A) (B) (C) (D)
10. (A) (B) (C) (D)
11. (A) (B) (C) (D)
12. (A) (B) (C) (D)
13. (A) (B) (C) (D)
14. (A) (B) (C) (D)
15. (A) (B) (C) (D)
16. (A) (B) (C) (D)
17. (A) (B) (C) (D)

18. (A) (B) (C) (D)
19. (A) (B) (C) (D)
20. (A) (B) (C) (D)
21. (A) (B) (C) (D)
22. (A) (B) (C) (D)
23. (A) (B) (C) (D)
24. (A) (B) (C) (D)
25. (A) (B) (C) (D)
26. (A) (B) (C) (D)
27. (A) (B) (C) (D)
28. (A) (B) (C) (D)
29. (A) (B) (C) (D)
30. (A) (B) (C) (D)
31. (A) (B) (C) (D)
32. (A) (B) (C) (D)
33. (A) (B) (C) (D)
34. (A) (B) (C) (D)

35. (A) (B) (C) (D)
36. (A) (B) (C) (D)
37. (A) (B) (C) (D)
38. (A) (B) (C) (D)
39. (A) (B) (C) (D)
40. (A) (B) (C) (D)
41. (A) (B) (C) (D)
42. (A) (B) (C) (D)
43. (A) (B) (C) (D)
44. (A) (B) (C) (D)
45. (A) (B) (C) (D)
46. (A) (B) (C) (D)
47. (A) (B) (C) (D)
48. (A) (B) (C) (D)
49. (A) (B) (C) (D)
50. (A) (B) (C) (D)

Mathematics

1. Ⓐ Ⓑ Ⓒ Ⓓ

2. Ⓐ Ⓑ Ⓒ Ⓓ

3. Ⓐ Ⓑ Ⓒ Ⓓ

4. Ⓐ Ⓑ Ⓒ Ⓓ

5. Ⓐ Ⓑ Ⓒ Ⓓ

6. Ⓐ Ⓑ Ⓒ Ⓓ

7. Ⓐ Ⓑ Ⓒ Ⓓ

8. Ⓐ Ⓑ Ⓒ Ⓓ

9. Ⓐ Ⓑ Ⓒ Ⓓ

10. Ⓐ Ⓑ Ⓒ Ⓓ

11. Ⓐ Ⓑ Ⓒ Ⓓ

12. Ⓐ Ⓑ Ⓒ Ⓓ

13. Ⓐ Ⓑ Ⓒ Ⓓ

14. Ⓐ Ⓑ Ⓒ Ⓓ

15. Ⓐ Ⓑ Ⓒ Ⓓ

16. Ⓐ Ⓑ Ⓒ Ⓓ

17. Ⓐ Ⓑ Ⓒ Ⓓ

18. Ⓐ Ⓑ Ⓒ Ⓓ

19. Ⓐ Ⓑ Ⓒ Ⓓ

20. Ⓐ Ⓑ Ⓒ Ⓓ

21. Ⓐ Ⓑ Ⓒ Ⓓ

22. Ⓐ Ⓑ Ⓒ Ⓓ

23. Ⓐ Ⓑ Ⓒ Ⓓ

24. Ⓐ Ⓑ Ⓒ Ⓓ

25. Ⓐ Ⓑ Ⓒ Ⓓ

26. Ⓐ Ⓑ Ⓒ Ⓓ

27. Ⓐ Ⓑ Ⓒ Ⓓ

28. Ⓐ Ⓑ Ⓒ Ⓓ

29. Ⓐ Ⓑ Ⓒ Ⓓ

30. Ⓐ Ⓑ Ⓒ Ⓓ

31. Ⓐ Ⓑ Ⓒ Ⓓ

32. Ⓐ Ⓑ Ⓒ Ⓓ

33. Ⓐ Ⓑ Ⓒ Ⓓ

34. Ⓐ Ⓑ Ⓒ Ⓓ

35. Ⓐ Ⓑ Ⓒ Ⓓ

36. Ⓐ Ⓑ Ⓒ Ⓓ

37. Ⓐ Ⓑ Ⓒ Ⓓ

38. Ⓐ Ⓑ Ⓒ Ⓓ

39. Ⓐ Ⓑ Ⓒ Ⓓ

40. Ⓐ Ⓑ Ⓒ Ⓓ

41. Ⓐ Ⓑ Ⓒ Ⓓ

42. Ⓐ Ⓑ Ⓒ Ⓓ

43. Ⓐ Ⓑ Ⓒ Ⓓ

44. Ⓐ Ⓑ Ⓒ Ⓓ

45. Ⓐ Ⓑ Ⓒ Ⓓ

46. Ⓐ Ⓑ Ⓒ Ⓓ

47. Ⓐ Ⓑ Ⓒ Ⓓ

48. Ⓐ Ⓑ Ⓒ Ⓓ

49. Ⓐ Ⓑ Ⓒ Ⓓ

50. Ⓐ Ⓑ Ⓒ Ⓓ

English Grammar

1. (A) (B) (C) (D)

2. (A) (B) (C) (D)

3. (A) (B) (C) (D)

4. (A) (B) (C) (D)

5. (A) (B) (C) (D)

6. (A) (B) (C) (D)

7. (A) (B) (C) (D)

8. (A) (B) (C) (D)

9. (A) (B) (C) (D)

10. (A) (B) (C) (D)

11. (A) (B) (C) (D)

12. (A) (B) (C) (D)

13. (A) (B) (C) (D)

14. (A) (B) (C) (D)

15. (A) (B) (C) (D)

16. (A) (B) (C) (D)

17. (A) (B) (C) (D)

18. (A) (B) (C) (D)

19. (A) (B) (C) (D)

20. (A) (B) (C) (D)

21. (A) (B) (C) (D)

22. (A) (B) (C) (D)

23. (A) (B) (C) (D)

24. (A) (B) (C) (D)

25. (A) (B) (C) (D)

26. (A) (B) (C) (D)

27. (A) (B) (C) (D)

28. (A) (B) (C) (D)

29. (A) (B) (C) (D)

30. (A) (B) (C) (D)

31. (A) (B) (C) (D)

32. (A) (B) (C) (D)

33. (A) (B) (C) (D)

34. (A) (B) (C) (D)

35. (A) (B) (C) (D)

36. (A) (B) (C) (D)

37. (A) (B) (C) (D)

38. (A) (B) (C) (D)

39. (A) (B) (C) (D)

40. (A) (B) (C) (D)

41. (A) (B) (C) (D)

42. (A) (B) (C) (D)

43. (A) (B) (C) (D)

44. (A) (B) (C) (D)

45. (A) (B) (C) (D)

46. (A) (B) (C) (D)

47. (A) (B) (C) (D)

48. (A) (B) (C) (D)

49. (A) (B) (C) (D)

50. (A) (B) (C) (D)

Vocabulary

1. Ⓐ Ⓑ Ⓒ Ⓓ
2. Ⓐ Ⓑ Ⓒ Ⓓ
3. Ⓐ Ⓑ Ⓒ Ⓓ
4. Ⓐ Ⓑ Ⓒ Ⓓ
5. Ⓐ Ⓑ Ⓒ Ⓓ
6. Ⓐ Ⓑ Ⓒ Ⓓ
7. Ⓐ Ⓑ Ⓒ Ⓓ
8. Ⓐ Ⓑ Ⓒ Ⓓ
9. Ⓐ Ⓑ Ⓒ Ⓓ
10. Ⓐ Ⓑ Ⓒ Ⓓ
11. Ⓐ Ⓑ Ⓒ Ⓓ
12. Ⓐ Ⓑ Ⓒ Ⓓ
13. Ⓐ Ⓑ Ⓒ Ⓓ
14. Ⓐ Ⓑ Ⓒ Ⓓ
15. Ⓐ Ⓑ Ⓒ Ⓓ
16. Ⓐ Ⓑ Ⓒ Ⓓ
17. Ⓐ Ⓑ Ⓒ Ⓓ

18. Ⓐ Ⓑ Ⓒ Ⓓ
19. Ⓐ Ⓑ Ⓒ Ⓓ
20. Ⓐ Ⓑ Ⓒ Ⓓ
21. Ⓐ Ⓑ Ⓒ Ⓓ
22. Ⓐ Ⓑ Ⓒ Ⓓ
23. Ⓐ Ⓑ Ⓒ Ⓓ
24. Ⓐ Ⓑ Ⓒ Ⓓ
25. Ⓐ Ⓑ Ⓒ Ⓓ
26. Ⓐ Ⓑ Ⓒ Ⓓ
27. Ⓐ Ⓑ Ⓒ Ⓓ
28. Ⓐ Ⓑ Ⓒ Ⓓ
29. Ⓐ Ⓑ Ⓒ Ⓓ
30. Ⓐ Ⓑ Ⓒ Ⓓ
31. Ⓐ Ⓑ Ⓒ Ⓓ
32. Ⓐ Ⓑ Ⓒ Ⓓ
33. Ⓐ Ⓑ Ⓒ Ⓓ
34. Ⓐ Ⓑ Ⓒ Ⓓ

35. Ⓐ Ⓑ Ⓒ Ⓓ
36. Ⓐ Ⓑ Ⓒ Ⓓ
37. Ⓐ Ⓑ Ⓒ Ⓓ
38. Ⓐ Ⓑ Ⓒ Ⓓ
39. Ⓐ Ⓑ Ⓒ Ⓓ
40. Ⓐ Ⓑ Ⓒ Ⓓ
41. Ⓐ Ⓑ Ⓒ Ⓓ
42. Ⓐ Ⓑ Ⓒ Ⓓ
43. Ⓐ Ⓑ Ⓒ Ⓓ
44. Ⓐ Ⓑ Ⓒ Ⓓ
45. Ⓐ Ⓑ Ⓒ Ⓓ
46. Ⓐ Ⓑ Ⓒ Ⓓ
47. Ⓐ Ⓑ Ⓒ Ⓓ
48. Ⓐ Ⓑ Ⓒ Ⓓ
49. Ⓐ Ⓑ Ⓒ Ⓓ
50. Ⓐ Ⓑ Ⓒ Ⓓ

Science

1. (A) (B) (C) (D)   21. (A) (B) (C) (D)   41. (A) (B) (C) (D)   61. (A) (B) (C) (D)

2. (A) (B) (C) (D)   22. (A) (B) (C) (D)   42. (A) (B) (C) (D)   62. (A) (B) (C) (D)

3. (A) (B) (C) (D)   23. (A) (B) (C) (D)   43. (A) (B) (C) (D)   63. (A) (B) (C) (D)

4. (A) (B) (C) (D)   24. (A) (B) (C) (D)   44. (A) (B) (C) (D)   64. (A) (B) (C) (D)

5. (A) (B) (C) (D)   25. (A) (B) (C) (D)   45. (A) (B) (C) (D)   65. (A) (B) (C) (D)

6. (A) (B) (C) (D)   26. (A) (B) (C) (D)   46. (A) (B) (C) (D)   66. (A) (B) (C) (D)

7. (A) (B) (C) (D)   27. (A) (B) (C) (D)   47. (A) (B) (C) (D)   67. (A) (B) (C) (D)

8. (A) (B) (C) (D)   28. (A) (B) (C) (D)   48. (A) (B) (C) (D)   68. (A) (B) (C) (D)

9. (A) (B) (C) (D)   29. (A) (B) (C) (D)   49. (A) (B) (C) (D)   69. (A) (B) (C) (D)

10. (A) (B) (C) (D)   30. (A) (B) (C) (D)   50. (A) (B) (C) (D)   70. (A) (B) (C) (D)

11. (A) (B) (C) (D)   31. (A) (B) (C) (D)   51. (A) (B) (C) (D)   71. (A) (B) (C) (D)

12. (A) (B) (C) (D)   32. (A) (B) (C) (D)   52. (A) (B) (C) (D)   72. (A) (B) (C) (D)

13. (A) (B) (C) (D)   33. (A) (B) (C) (D)   53. (A) (B) (C) (D)   73. (A) (B) (C) (D)

14. (A) (B) (C) (D)   34. (A) (B) (C) (D)   54. (A) (B) (C) (D)   74. (A) (B) (C) (D)

15. (A) (B) (C) (D)   35. (A) (B) (C) (D)   55. (A) (B) (C) (D)   75. (A) (B) (C) (D)

16. (A) (B) (C) (D)   36. (A) (B) (C) (D)   56. (A) (B) (C) (D)   76. (A) (B) (C) (D)

17. (A) (B) (C) (D)   37. (A) (B) (C) (D)   57. (A) (B) (C) (D)   77. (A) (B) (C) (D)

18. (A) (B) (C) (D)   38. (A) (B) (C) (D)   58. (A) (B) (C) (D)   78. (A) (B) (C) (D)

19. (A) (B) (C) (D)   39. (A) (B) (C) (D)   59. (A) (B) (C) (D)   79. (A) (B) (C) (D)

20. (A) (B) (C) (D)   40. (A) (B) (C) (D)   60. (A) (B) (C) (D)   80. (A) (B) (C) (D)

Anatomy and Physiology

1. (A) (B) (C) (D)   11. (A) (B) (C) (D)   21. (A) (B) (C) (D)

2. (A) (B) (C) (D)   12. (A) (B) (C) (D)   22. (A) (B) (C) (D)

3. (A) (B) (C) (D)   13. (A) (B) (C) (D)   23. (A) (B) (C) (D)

4. (A) (B) (C) (D)   14. (A) (B) (C) (D)   24. (A) (B) (C) (D)

5. (A) (B) (C) (D)   15. (A) (B) (C) (D)   25. (A) (B) (C) (D)

6. (A) (B) (C) (D)   16. (A) (B) (C) (D)

7. (A) (B) (C) (D)   17. (A) (B) (C) (D)

8. (A) (B) (C) (D)   18. (A) (B) (C) (D)

9. (A) (B) (C) (D)   19. (A) (B) (C) (D)

10. (A) (B) (C) (D)   20. (A) (B) (C) (D)

Section I - Reading Comprehension

Questions 1 - 4 refer to the following passage.

The Respiratory System

The respiratory system's function is to allow oxygen exchange through all parts of the body. The anatomy or structure of the exchange system, and the uses of the exchanged gases, varies depending on the organism. In humans and other mammals, for example, the anatomical features of the respiratory system include airways, lungs, and the respiratory muscles. Molecules of oxygen and carbon dioxide are passively exchanged, by diffusion, between the gaseous external environment and the blood. This exchange process occurs in the alveolar region of the lungs.

Other animals, such as insects, have respiratory systems with very simple anatomical features, and in amphibians even the skin plays a vital role in gas exchange. Plants also have respiratory systems but the direction of gas exchange can be opposite to that of animals.

The respiratory system can also be divided into physiological, or functional, zones. These include the conducting zone (the region for gas transport from the outside atmosphere to just above the alveoli), the transitional zone, and the respiratory zone (the alveolar region where gas exchange occurs). [12]

1. What can we infer from the first paragraph in this passage?

   a.   Human and mammal respiratory systems are the same.

   b.   The lungs are an important part of the respiratory system.

   c.   The respiratory system varies in different mammals.

   d.   Oxygen and carbon dioxide are passive exchanged by the respiratory system.

2. What is the process by which molecules of oxygen and carbon dioxide are passively exchanged?

    a. Transfusion

    b. Affusion

    c. Diffusion

    d. Respiratory confusion

3. What organ plays an important role in gas exchange in amphibians?

    a. The skin

    b. The lungs

    c. The gills

    d. The mouth

4. What are the three physiological zones of the respiratory system?

    a. Conducting, transitional, respiratory zones

    b. Redacting, transitional, circulatory zones

    c. Conducting, circulatory, inhibiting zones

    d. Transitional, inhibiting, conducting zones

Questions 5 - 8 refer to the following passage.

ABC Electric Warranty

ABC Electric Company warrants that its products are free from defects in material and workmanship.- Subject to the conditions and limitations set forth below, ABC Electric will, at its option, either repair or replace any part of its products that prove defective due to improper workmanship or materials.

This limited warranty does not cover any damage to the product from improper installation, accident, abuse, misuse, natural disaster, insufficient or excessive electrical supply, abnormal mechanical or environmental conditions, or any unauthorized disassembly, repair, or modification.

This limited warranty also does not apply to any product on which the original identification information has been altered, or removed, has not been handled or packaged correctly, or has been sold as second-hand.

This limited warranty covers only repair, replacement, refund or credit for defective ABC Electric products, as provided above.

5. I tried to repair my ABC Electric blender, but could not, so can I get it repaired under this warranty?

    a.   Yes, the warranty still covers the blender.

    b.   No, the warranty does not cover the blender.

    c.   Uncertain. ABC Electric may or may not cover repairs under this warranty.

6. My ABC Electric fan is not working. Will ABC Electric provide a new one or repair this one?

    a. ABC Electric will repair my fan

    b. ABC Electric will replace my fan

    c. ABC Electric could either replace or repair my fan or I can request either a replacement or a repair.

7. My stove was damaged in a flood. Does this warranty cover my stove?

    a. Yes, it is covered.

    b. No, it is not covered.

    c. It may or may not be covered.

    d. ABC Electric will decide if it is covered.

8. Which of the following is an example of improper workmanship?

    a. Missing parts

    b. Defective parts

    c. Scratches on the front

    d. None of the above

Questions 9 – 12 refer to the following passage.

Mythology

The main characters in myths are usually gods or supernatural heroes. As sacred stories, rulers and priests have traditionally endorsed their myths and as a result, myths have a close link with religion and politics. In the society where a myth originates, the natives believe the myth is a true account of the remote past. In fact, many societies have two categories of traditional narrative—(1) "true stories," or myths, and (2) "false stories," or fables.

Myths generally take place during a primordial age, when the world was still young, prior to achieving its current form. These stories explain how the world gained its current form and why the culture developed its customs, institutions, and taboos. Closely related to myth are legend and folktale. Myths, legends, and folktales are different types of traditional stories. Unlike myths, folktales can take place at any time and any place, and the natives do not usually consider them true or sacred. Legends, on the other hand, are similar to myths in that many people have traditionally considered them true. Legends take place in a more recent time, when the world was much as it is today. In addition, legends generally feature humans as their main characters, whereas myths have superhuman characters. [13]

9. We can infer from this passage that

a. Folktales took place in a time far past, before civilization covered the earth

b. Humankind uses myth to explain how the world was created

c. Myths revolve around gods or supernatural beings; the local community usually accepts these stories as not true

d. The only difference between a myth and a legend is the time setting of the story

10. The main purpose of this passage is

a. To distinguish between many types of traditional stories, and explain the back-ground of some traditional story categories

b. To determine whether myths and legends might be true accounts of history

c. To show the importance of folktales how these traditional stories made life more bearable in harder times

d. None of the Above

11. How are folktales different from myths?

a. Folktales and myth are the same

b. Folktales are not true and generally not sacred and take place anytime

c. Myths are not true and generally not sacred and take place anytime

d. Folktales explained the formation of the world and myths do not

12. How are legends and myth similar?

a. Many people believe legends and myths are true, myths take place in modern day, and legends are about ordinary people

b. Many people believe legends and myths are true, legends take place in modern day, and legends are about ordinary people

c. Many people believe legends and myths are true, legends take place in modern day, and myths are about ordinary people

d. Many people believe legends and myths are not true, legends take place in mod-ern day, and legends are about ordinary people

Questions 13 - 16 refer to the following passage.

Myths, Legend and Folklore

Cultural historians draw a distinction between myth, legend and folktale simply as a way to group traditional stories. However, in many cultures, drawing a sharp line between myths and legends is not that simple. Instead of dividing their traditional stories into myths, legends, and folktales, some cultures divide them into two categories. The first category roughly corresponds to folktales, and the second is one that combines myths and legends. Similarly, we cannot always separate myths from folktales. One society might consider a story true, making it a myth. Another society may believe the story is fiction, which makes it a folktale. In fact, when a myth loses its status as part of a religious system, it often takes on traits more typical of folktales, with its formerly divine characters now appearing as human heroes, giants, or fairies. Myth, legend, and folktale are only a few of the categories of traditional stories. Other categories include anecdotes and some kinds of jokes. Traditional stories, in turn, are only one category within the larger category of folklore, which also includes items such as gestures, costumes, and music. [13]

13. The main idea of this passage is that

a. Myths, fables, and folktales are not the same thing, and each describes a specific type of story.

b. Traditional stories can be categorized in different ways by different people.

c. Cultures use myths for religious purposes, and when this is no longer true, the people forget and discard these myths.

d. Myths can never become folk tales, because one is true, and the other is false.

14. The terms myth and legend are

a. Categories that are synonymous with true and false.

b. Categories that group traditional stories according to certain characteristics.

c. Interchangeable, because both terms mean a story that is passed down from generation to generation.

d. Meant to distinguish between a story that involves a hero and a cultural message and a story meant only to entertain.

15. Traditional story categories not only include myths and legends, but

a. Can also include gestures, since some cultures passed these down before the written and spoken word.

b. In addition, folklore refers to stories involving fables and fairy tales.

c. These story categories can also include folk music and traditional dress.

d. Traditional stories themselves are a part of the larger category of folklore, which may also include costumes, gestures, and music.

16. This passage shows that

a. There is a distinct difference between a myth and a legend, although both are folktales.

b. Myths are folktales, but folktales are not myths.

c. Myths, legends, and folktales play an important part in tradition and the past, and are a rich and colorful part of history.

d. Most cultures consider myths to be true.

Questions 17 - 19 refer to the following passage.

Insects

Humans regard certain insects as pests and attempt to control them with insecticides and many other techniques. Some insects damage crops by feeding on sap, leaves or fruits, a few bite humans and livestock, alive and dead, to feed on blood and some are capable of transmitting diseases to humans, pets and live-stock. Many other insects are considered ecologically beneficial and a few provide direct economic benefit. Silkworms and bees, for example, have been domesticated for the production of silk and honey, respectively. [14]

17. How do humans control insects?

a. By training them

b. Using insecticides and other techniques

c. In many different ways

d. Humans do not control insects

18. Why do humans control insects?

a. Because they do not like them

b. Because they damage crops

c. Because they damage buildings

d. Because they damage the soil

19. How do insects damage crops?

   a. By feeding on crops
   b. By transmitting disease
   c. By laying eggs on crops
   d. None of the above

Questions 20 - 23 refer to the following passage.

Was Dr. Seuss A Real Doctor?

A favorite author for over 100 years, Theodor Seuss Geisel was born on March 2, 1902. Today, we celebrate the birthday of the famous "Dr. Seuss" by hosting Read Across America events throughout the month of March. School children around the country celebrate the "Doctor's" birthday by making hats, giving presentations and holding read aloud circles featuring some of Dr. Seuss' most famous books.

But who was Dr. Seuss? Did he go to medical school? Where was his office? You may be surprised to know that Theodor Seuss Geisel was not a medical doctor at all. He took on the nickname Dr. Seuss when he became a noted children's book author. He earned the nickname because people said his books were "as good as medicine." All these years later, his nickname has lasted and he is known as Dr. Seuss all across the world.
Think back to when you were a young child. Did you ever want to try "green eggs and ham."? Did you try to "Hop on Pop"? Do you remember learning about the environment from a creature called The Lorax? Of course, you must recall one of Seuss' most famous characters; that green Grinch who stole Christmas. These stories were all written by Dr. Seuss and featured his signature rhyming words and letters. They also featured made up words to enhance his rhyme scheme and even though many of his characters were made up, they sure seem real to us today.

And what of his "signature" book, The Cat in the Hat? You must remember that cat and Thing One and Thing Two from your childhood. Did you know that in the early 1950's there was a growing concern in America that children were not becoming avid readers? This was, book publishers thought, because children found that books dull and uninteresting. An intelligent publisher sent Dr. Seuss a book of words that he thought all children should learn as young readers. Dr. Seuss wrote his famous story The Cat in the Hat, using those words. We can see, over the decades, just how much influence his writing has had on very young children. That is why we celebrate this doctor's birthday each March.

20. What does the word "avid" mean in the last paragraph?

    a. Good

    b. Interested

    c. Slow

    d. Fast

21. What can we infer from the statement " His books were like medicine"?

    a. His books made people feel better

    b. His books were in doctor's office waiting rooms

    c. His books took away fevers

    d. His books left a funny taste in readers' mouths.

22. Why is the publisher in the last paragraph called "intelligent?"

    a. The publisher knew how to read.

    b. The publisher knew kids did not like to read.

    c. The publisher knew Dr. Seuss would be able to create a book that sold well.

    d. The publisher knew that Dr. Seuss would be able to write a book that would get young children interested in reading.

23. The theme of this passage is

a. Dr. Seuss was not a doctor.

b. Dr. Seuss influenced the lives of generations of young children.

c. Dr. Seuss wrote rhyming books.

d. Dr. Suess' birthday is a good day to read a book.

Questions 24 - 27 refer to the following passage.

Passage 7 – Trees

With an estimated 100,000 species, trees represent 25 percent of all living plant species. Most tree species grow in tropical regions of the world and many of these areas have not been surveyed by botanists, making species diversity poorly understood. The earliest trees were tree ferns and horsetails, which grew in forests in the Carboniferous period. Tree ferns still survive, but the only surviving horsetails are no longer in tree form. Later, in the Triassic period, conifers and ginkgos, appeared, followed by flowering plants after that in the Cretaceous period. [15]

24. Do botanists understand the number of tree species?

a. Yes, botanists know exactly how many tree species exit.

b. No, the species diversity is not well understood.

c. Yes, botanists have a general idea.

d. No, botanists have no idea.

25. Where do most trees species grow?

a. Most tree species grow in tropical regions.

b. There is no one area where most tree species grow.

c. Tree species grow in 25% of the world.

d. There are 100,000 tree species.

26. What tree(s) survived from the Carboniferous period?

    a. 25% of all trees

    b. Horsetails

    c. Conifers

    d. Tree Ferns

27. Choose the correct list below, ranked from oldest to youngest trees.

    a. Flowering plants, conifers and ginkgos, tree ferns and horsetails.

    b. Tree ferns and horsetails, conifers and ginkgos, flowering plants.

    c. Tree ferns and horsetails, flowering plants, conifers and ginkgos.

    d. Conifers and ginkgos, tree ferns and horsetails, flowering plants.

Questions 28 - 29 refer to the following passage.

Lowest Price Guarantee

Get it for less. Guaranteed!

ABC Electric will beat any advertised price by 10% of the difference.

    1) If you find a lower advertised price, we will beat it by 10% of the difference.

    2) If you find a lower advertised price within 30 days* of your purchase we will beat it by 10% of the difference.

    3) If our own price is reduced within 30 days* of your purchase, bring in your receipt and we will refund the difference.

*14 days for computers, monitors, printers, laptops, tablets, cellular & wireless devices, home security products, projectors, camcorders, digital cameras, radar detectors, portable DVD players, DJ and pro-audio equipment, and air conditioners.

28. I bought a radar detector 15 days ago and saw an ad for the same model only cheaper. Can I get 10% of the difference refunded?

 a. Yes. Since it is less than 30 days, you can get 10% of the difference refunded.

 b. No. Since it is more than 14 days, you cannot get 10% of the difference re-funded.

 c. It depends on the cashier.

 d. Yes. You can get the difference refunded.

29. I bought a flat-screen TV for $500 10 days ago and found an advertisement for the same TV, at another store, on sale for $400. How much will ABC refund under this guarantee?

 a. $100

 b. $110

 c. $10

 d. $400

Questions 30 - 33 refer to the following passage.

Who Was Anne Frank?

You may have heard mention of the word Holocaust in your History or English classes. The Holocaust took place from 1939-1945. It was an attempt by the Nazi party to purify the human race, by eliminating Jews, Gypsies, Catholics, homosexuals and others they deemed inferior to their "perfect" Aryan race. The Nazis used Concentration Camps, which were sometimes used as Death Camps, to exterminate the people they held in the camps. One of the saddest facts about the Holocaust was the over one million children under the age of sixteen died in a Nazi concentration camp.

Just a few weeks before World War II was over, Anne Frank was one of those children to die.

Before the Nazi party began its persecution of the Jews, Anne Frank had a happy live. She was born in June of 1929. In June of 1942, for her 13th birthday, she was given a simple present which would go onto impact the lives of millions of people around the world. That gift was a small red diary that she called Kitty. This diary was to become Anne's most treasured possession when she and her family hid from the Nazi's in a secret annex above her father's office building in Amsterdam.

For 25 months, Anne, her sister Margot, her parents, another family, and an elderly Jewish dentist hid from the Nazis in this tiny annex. They were never permitted to go outside and their food and supplies were brought to them by Miep Gies and her husband, who did not believe in the Nazi persecution of the Jews. It was a very difficult life for young Anne and she used Kitty as an outlet to describe her life in hiding.

After 2 years, Anne and her family were betrayed and arrested by the Nazis. To this day, nobody is exactly sure who betrayed the Frank family and the other annex residents. Anne, her mother, and her sister were separated from Otto Frank, Anne's father. Then, Anne and Margot were separated from their mother. In March of 1945, Margot Frank died of starvation in a Concentration Camp. A few days later, at the age of 15, Anne Frank died of typhus. Of all the people who hid in the Annex, only Otto Frank survived the Holocaust.

Otto Frank returned to the Annex after World War II. It was there that he found Kitty, filled with Anne's thoughts and feelings about being a persecuted Jewish girl. Otto Frank had Anne's diary published in 1947 and it has remained continuously in print ever since. Today, the diary has been published in over 55 languages and more than 24 million copies have been sold around the world. The Diary of Anne Frank tells the story of a brave young woman who tried to see the good in all people.

30. From the context clues in the passage, the word Annex most nearly means?

    a. Attic

    b. Bedroom

    c. Basement

    d. Kitchen

31. Why do you think Anne's diary has been published in 55 languages?

    a. So everyone could understand it.

    b. So people around the world could learn more about the horrors of the Holocaust.

    c. Because Anne was Jewish but hid in Amsterdam and died in Germany.

    d. Because Otto Frank spoke many languages.

32. From the description of Anne and Margot's deaths in the passage, what can we assume typhus is?

    a. The same as starving to death.

    b. An infection the Germans gave to Anne.

    c. A disease Anne caught in the concentration camp.

    d. Poison gas used by the Germans to kill Anne.

33. In the third paragraph, what does the word outlet most nearly mean?

    a. A place to plug things into the wall

    b. A store where Miep bought cheap supplies for the Frank family

    c. A hiding space similar to an Annex

    d. A place where Anne could express her private thoughts.

Questions 34 - 37 refer to the following passage.

Passage 10 - The Circulatory System

The circulatory system is an organ system that passes nutrients (such as amino acids and electrolytes), gases, hormones, and blood cells to and from cells in the body to help fight diseases and help stabilize body temperature and pH levels.

The circulatory system may be seen strictly as a blood distribution network, but some consider the circulatory system as composed of the cardiovascular system, which distributes blood, and the lymphatic system, which distributes lymph. While humans, as well as other vertebrates, have a closed cardiovascular system (meaning that the blood never leaves the network of arteries, veins and capillaries), some invertebrate groups have an open cardiovascular system. The most primitive animal phyla lack circulatory systems. The lymphatic system, on the other hand, is an open system.

Two types of fluids move through the circulatory system: blood and lymph. The blood, heart, and blood vessels form the cardiovascular system. The lymph, lymph nodes, and lymph vessels form the lymphatic system. The cardiovascular system and the lymphatic system collectively make up the circulatory system.

The main components of the human cardiovascular system are the heart and the blood vessels. It includes: the pulmonary circulation, a "loop" through the lungs where blood is oxygenated; and the systemic circulation, a "loop" through the rest of the body to provide oxygenated blood. An average adult contains five to six quarts (roughly 4.7 to 5.7 liters) of blood, which consists of plasma, red blood cells, white blood cells, and platelets. Also, the digestive system works with the circulatory system to provide the nutrients the system needs to keep the heart pumping. [16]

34. What can we infer from the first paragraph?

a. An important purpose of the circulatory system is that of fighting diseases.

b. The most important function of the circulatory system is to give the person energy.

c. The least important function of the circulatory system is that of growing skin cells.

d. The entire purpose of the circulatory system is not known.

35. Do humans have an open or closed circulatory system?

a. Open

b. Closed

c. Usually open, though sometimes closed

d. Usually closed, though sometimes open

36. In addition to blood, what two components form the cardiovascular system?

a. The heart and the lungs

b. The lungs and the veins

c. The heart and the blood vessels

d. The blood vessels and the nerves

37. Which system, along with the circulatory system, helps provide nutrients to keep the human heart pumping?

a. The skeletal system

b. The digestive system

c. The immune system

d. The nervous system

Questions 38 - 41 refer to the following passage.

The Life of Helen Keller

Many people have heard of Helen Keller. She is famous because she was unable to see or hear, but learned to speak and read and went on to attend college and earn a degree. Her life is a very interesting story, one that she developed into an autobiography, which was then adapted into both a stage play and a movie. How did Helen Keller overcome her disabilities to become a famous woman?

Helen Keller was not born blind and deaf. When she was a small baby, she had a very high fever for several days. As a result of her sudden illness, baby Helen lost her eyesight and her hearing. Because she was so young when she went deaf and blind, Helen Keller never had any recollection of being able to see or hear. Since she could not hear, she could not learn to talk. Since she could not see, it was difficult for her to move around. For the first six years of her life, her world was very still and dark.

Imagine what Helen's childhood was like. She could not hear her mother's voice. She could not see the beauty of her parent's farm. She could not recognize who was giving her a hug, or a bath or even where her bedroom was each night. More sad, she could not communicate with her parents in any way. She could not express her feelings or tell them the things she wanted. It must have been a very sad childhood.

When Helen was six years old, her parents hired her a teacher named Anne Sullivan. Anne was a young woman who was almost blind. However, she could hear and she could read Braille, so she was a perfect teacher for young Helen. At first, Anne had a very hard time teaching Helen anything. She described her first impression of Helen as a "wild thing, not a child." Helen did not like Anne at first either. She bit and hit Anne when Anne tried to teach her. However, the two of them eventually came to have a great deal of love and respect.

Anne taught Helen to hear by putting her hands on peo-

ple's throats. She could feel the sounds that people made.
In time, Helen learned to feel what people said. Next, Anne
taught Helen to read Braille, which is a way that books are
written for the blind. Finally, Anne taught Helen to talk.
Although Helen did learn to talk, it was hard for anyone
but Anne to understand her.

As Helen grew older, she amazed people with her story.
She went to college and wrote books about her life. She
gave talks to the public, with Anne at her side, translating
her words. Today, both Anne Sullivan and Helen Keller are
famous women who are respected for their lives' work.

**38. Helen Keller could not see and hear and so, her big-
gest problem in childhood was her inability to do what?**

    a. Communicate

    b. Walk

    c. Play

    d. Eat

**39. Helen learned to hear by feeling the vibrations
people made when they spoke. What were these vibrations were felt through?**

    a. Mouth

    b. Throat

    c. Ears

    d. Lips

**40. From the passage, we can infer that Anne Sullivan
was a patient teacher. We can infer this because**

    a. Helen hit and bit her and Anne remained her
    teacher.

    b. Anne taught Helen to read only.

    c. Anne was hard of hearing too.

    d. Anne wanted to be a teacher.

41. Helen Keller learned to speak but Anne translated her words when she spoke in public. The reason Helen needed a translator was because

    a. Helen spoke another language.

    b. Helen's words were hard for people to understand.

    c. Helen spoke very quietly.

    d. Helen did not speak but only used sign language.

Questions 42 - 45 refer to the following passage.

Passage 12 - The Human Skeleton

The human skeleton consists of both fused and individual bones supported and supplemented by ligaments, tendons, muscles and cartilage. It serves as a scaffold which supports organs, anchors muscles, and protects organs such as the brain, lungs and heart. The biggest bone in the body is the femur in the upper leg, and the smallest is the stapes bone in the middle ear. In an adult, the skeleton comprises around 14% of the total body weight, and half of this weight is water.

Fused bones include the pelvis and the cranium. Not all bones are interconnected directly: There are three bones in each middle ear called the ossicles that articulate only with each other. The thyroid bone, which is located in the neck, and serves as the point of attachment for the tongue, does not articulate with any other bones in the body, being supported by muscles and ligaments.

There are 206 bones in the adult human skeleton, which varies between individuals and with age - newborn babies have over 270 bones, some of which fuse together. These bones are organized into a longitudinal axis, the axial skeleton, to which the appendicular skeleton is attached. [17]

42. What is the main idea of this passage?

a. The human skeleton is an important and complicated system of the body.

b. There are 206 bones in the typical human body.

c. In a child, the skeleton represents 14% of the body
weight.

d. Bones become more fragile as we age.

43. How many bones are located in the human middle ear?

a. 3

b. 2

c. 1

d. 0

44. Which of the following is not true about the number of bones in the human skeleton?

a. The typical skeleton has 206 bones.

b. The number of bones stays the same throughout
one's lifetime.

c. Newborn babies have about 270 bones.

d. As a baby grows older, some of its bones fuse together.

45. What is the appendicular skeleton attached to?

a. The exoskeleton.

b. The radial skeleton.

c. The rotating skeleton.

d. The axial skeleton.

Section II – Math

1. 8327 – 1278 =

   a. 7149

   b. 7209

   c. 6059

   d. 7049

2. 294 X 21 =

   a. 6017

   b. 6174

   c. 6728

   d. 5679

3. 1278 + 4920 =

   a. 6298

   b. 6108

   c. 6198

   d. 6098

4. 285 * 12 =

   a. 3420

   b. 3402

   c. 3024

   d. 2322

5. 4120 – 3216 =

   a. 903

   b. 804

   c. 904

   d. 1904

6. 2417 + 1004 =

   a. 3401

   b. 4321

   c. 3402

   d. 3421

7. 1440 ÷ 12 =

   a. 122

   b. 120

   c. 110

   d. 132

8. 2713 – 1308 =

   a. 1450

   b. 1445

   c. 1405

   d. 1455

9. It is known that $x^2 + 4x$ = 5. Then x can be

   a. 0

   b. -5

   c. 1

   d. Either (b) or (c)

10. (a + b)2 = 4ab. What is necessarily correct?

   a. a > b

   b. a < b

   c. a = b

   d. None of the Above

11. The sum of the digits of a 2-digit number is 12. If we switch the digits, the number will be greater than the initial one by 36. Find the initial number.

    a. 39

    b. 48

    c. 57

    d. 75

12. In a class of 83 students, 72 are present. What percent of student is absent?

    a. 12

    b. 13

    c. 14

    d. 15

13. Kate's father is 32 years older than Kate is. In 5 years, he will be five times older. How old is Kate?

    a. 2

    b. 3

    c. 5

    d. 6

14. If Lynn can type a page in p minutes, what portion of the page can she do in 5 minutes?

    a. 5/p

    b. p - 5

    c. p + 5

    d. p/5

15. If Sally can paint a house in 4 hours, and John can paint the same house in 6 hours, how long will it take for both of them to paint the house together?

    a. 2 hours and 24 minutes

    b. 3 hours and 12 minutes

    c. 3 hours and 44 minutes

    d. 4 hours and 10 minutes

16. Employees of a discount appliance store receive an additional 20% off the lowest price on any item. If an employee purchases a dishwasher during a 15% off sale, how much will he pay if the dishwasher originally cost $450?

    a. $280.90

    b. $287.00

    c. $292.50

    d. $306.00

17. The sale price of a car is $12,590, which is 20% off the original price. What is the original price?

    a. $14,310.40

    b. $14,990.90

    c. $15,108.00

    d. $15,737.50

18. A goat eats 214 kg. of hay in 60 days, while a cow eats the same amount in 15 days. How long will it take them to eat this hay together?

    a. 37.5

    b. 75

    c. 12

    d. 15

19. Express 25% as a fraction.

    a. 1/4

    b. 7/40

    c. 6/25

    d. 8/28

20. Express 125% as a decimal.

    a. .125

    b. 12.5

    c. 1.25

    d. 125

21. Solve for x: 30 is 40% of x

    a. 60

    b. 90

    c. 85

    d. 75

22. 12 ½% of x is equal to 50. Solve for x.

    a. 300

    b. 400

    c. 450

    d. 350

23. Express 24/56 as a reduced common fraction.

    a. 4/9

    b. 4/11

    c. 3/7

    d. 3/8

24. Express 87% as a decimal.

    a. .087

    b. 8.7

    c. .87

    d. 87

25. 60 is 75% of x. Solve for x.

    a. 80

    b. 90

    c. 75

    d. 70

26. 60% of x is 12. Solve for x.

    a. 18

    b. 15

    c. 25

    d. 20

27. Express 71/1000 as a decimal.

    a. .71

    b. .0071

    c. .071

    d. 7.1

28. 4.7 + .9 + .01 =

    a. 5.5

    b. 6.51

    c. 5.61

    d. 5.7

29. .33 × .59 =

    a. .1947

    b. 1.947

    c. .0197

    d. .1817

30. .84 ÷ .7 =

    a. .12

    b. 12

    c. .012

    d. 1.2

31. What number is in the ten thousandths place in 1.7389?

    a. 1

    b. 8

    c. 9

    d. 3

32. .87 - .48 =

    a. .39

    b. .49

    c. .41

    d. .37

33. The physician ordered 100 mg Ibuprofen/kg of body weight; on hand is 230 mg/tablet. The child weighs 50 lb. How many tablets will you give?

    a. 10 tablets

    b. 5 tablets

    c. 1 tablet

    d. 12 tablets

34. The physician ordered 1,000 units of heparin; 5,000 U/mL is on hand. How many milliliters will you give?

    a. 0.002 ml

    b. 0.2 ml

    c. 0.02 ml

    d. 2 ml

35. Simplify 4^3

    a. 20

    b. 32

    c. 64

    d. 108

36. The physician ordered 5 mL of Capacitate; 15 mL/tsp is on hand. How many teaspoons will you give?

    a. 0.05 tsp

    b. 0.03 tsp

    c. 0.5 tsp

    d. 0.3 tsp

37. The physician orders 70 mg morphine sulphate; 1 g/mL is on hand. How many mL will you give?

    a. 0.05 ml

    b. 0.07 ml

    c. 0.04 ml

    d. 0.007 ml

38. The physician ordered 200 mg amoxicillin. The pharmacy stocks amoxicillin 400 mg per tsp. How many teaspoons will you give?

    a. 0.55 tsp

    b. 0.25 tsp

    c. 0.5 tsp

    d. 0.05 tsp

39. The physician ordered 600 mg ibuprofen po; the office stocks 200 mg per tablet. How many tablets will you give?

    a. 3.5 tablets

    b. 2 tablets

    c. 5 tablets

    d. 3 tablets

40. The manager of a weaving factory estimates that if 10 machines run on 100% efficiency for 8 hours, they will produce 1450 meters of cloth. However, due to some technical problems, 4 machines run of 95% efficiency and the remaining 6 at 90% efficiency. How many meters of cloth can these machines will produce in 8 hours?

    a. 1334 meters

    b. 1310 meters

    c. 1300 meters

    d. 1285 meters

41. Convert 60 feet to inches.

    a. 700 inches

    b. 600 inches

    c. 720 inches

    d. 1,800 inches

42. Convert 25 centimeters to millimeters.

    a. 250 millimeters

    b. 7.5 millimeters

    c. 5 millimeters

    d. 2.5 millimeters

43. Convert 100 millimeters to centimeters.

    a. 10 centimeters

    b. 1,000 centimeters

    c. 1100 centimeters

    d. 50 centimeters

44. Convert 3 gallons to quarts.

    a. 15 quarts

    b. 6 quarts

    c. 12 quarts

    d. 32 quarts

45. 2000 mm. =

    a. 2 m

    b. 200 m

    c. 0.002 m

    d. 0.02 m

46. 0.05 ml. =

    a. 50 liters

    b. 0.00005 liters

    c. 5 liters

    d. 0.0005 liters

47. 30 mg is the same mass as:

    a. 0.0003 kg.

    b. 0.03 grams

    c. 300 decigrams

    d. 0.3 grams

48. 0.101 mm. =

   a. .0101 cm

   b. 1.01 cm

   c. 0.00101 cm

   d. 10.10 cm

49. Smith and Simon are playing a card game. Smith will win if a card drawn from a deck of 52 is either 7 or a diamond, and Simon will win if the drawn card is an even number. Which statement is more likely to be correct?

   a. Smith will win more games.

   b. Simon will win more games.

   c. They have same winning probability.

   d. A decision cannot be made from the provided data.

50. How much water can be stored in a cylindrical container 5 meters in diameter and 12 meters high?

   a. 223.65 m^3

   b. 235.65 m^3

   c. 240.65 m^3

   d. 252.65 m^3

Section III – English Grammar

Fill in the blank.

1. Elaine promised to bring the camera _____ at the mall yesterday.

    a. by me

    b. with me

    c. at me

    d. to me

2. Last night, he _____ the sleeping bag down beside my mattress.

    a. lay

    b. laid

    c. lain

    d. has laid

3. I would have bought the shirt for you if _____.

    a. I had known you liked it.

    b. I have known you liked it.

    c. I would know you liked it.

    d. I know you liked it.

4. Many believers still hope _____ proof of the existence of ghosts.

    a. two find

    b. to find

    c. to found

    d. to have been found

5. All of the people at the school, including the teachers and _____ were glad when summer break came.

    a. students:

    b. students,

    c. students;

    d. students

6. Choose the sentence with the correct grammar.

    a. Each player gets a locker to keep their personal things.

    b. Each player gets a locker to keep his personal things.

    c. Each player gets a locker to keep our personal things.

    d. None of the above.

7. If he _____ the textbook like he was supposed to, he would have known what was on the test.

    a. will have read

    b. shouldn't have read

    c. would have read

    d. had read

8. Following the tornado, telephone poles _____ all over the street.

    a. laid

    b. lied

    c. were lying

    d. were laying

9. In Edgar Allen Poe's _____ Edgar Allen Poe describes a man with a guilty conscience.

    a. short story, "The Tell-Tale Heart,"

    b. short story The Tell-Tale Heart,

    c. short story, The Tell-Tale Heart

    d. short story. "the Tell-Tale Heart,"

10. Billboards are considered an important part of advertising for big business, _____ by their critics.

    a. but, an eyesore;

    b. but, " an eyesore,"

    c. but an eyesore

    d. but-an eyesore-

11. I can never remember how to use those two common words, "sell," meaning to trade a product for money, or _____ meaning an event where products are traded for less money than usual.

    a. sale-

    b. "sale,"

    c. "sale

    d. "to sale,"

12. The class just finished reading _____ a short story by Carl Stephenson about a plantation owner's battle with army ants.

    a. "Leinengen versus the Ants,"

    b. Leinengen versus the Ants,

    c. "Leinengen versus the Ants,"

    d. Leinengen versus the Ants

13. After the car was fixed, it _____ again.

    a. ran good

    b. ran well

    c. would have run well

    d. ran more well

14. "Where does the sun go during the _____ asked little Kathy.

    a. night,"

    b. night"?,

    c. night,?"

    d. night?"

15. Choose the best revision of the sentence.

When I was a child, my mother taught me to say thank you, holding the door open for other, and cover my mouth when yawning or coughing.

    a. When I was a child, my mother teaching me to say thank you, to hold the door open for others, and cover my mouth when yawning or coughing.

    b. When I was a child, my mother taught me say thank you, to hold the door open for others, and to covering my mouth when yawning or coughing.

    c. When I was a child, my mother taught me saying thank you, holding the door open for others, and to cover my mouth when yawning or coughing.

    d. When I was a child, my mother taught me to say thank you, hold the door open for others, and cover my mouth when yawning or coughing.

16. Choose the best revision of the sentence.

Mother is talking to a man that wants to hire her to be a receptionist.

a. Mother is talking to a man who wants to hire her to be a receptionist.

b. Mother is talked to a man who wants to hire her to be a receptionist.

c. Mother is talking to a man who wants to her. To be a receptionist.

d. Mother is talking to a man hiring her who to be a receptionist.

17. Choose the best revision of the sentence.

Those comic books, which was for sale at the magazine shop, are now quite valuable.

a. Those comics books which were for sale, at the magazine shop are now quite valuable.

b. Those comic books, which were for sale at the magazine, shop, are now quite valuable.

c. Those comic books, which were for sale at the magazine shop, are now, quite valuable

d. Those comic books, which were for sale at the magazine shop, are now quite valuable.

18. Choose the best revision of the sentence.

If you want to sell your car, it's important being honest with the buyer.

a. If you want to sell your car, being honest with the buyer is important.

b. If you want to sell your car, to be honest with the buyer is important.

c. If you wanting to sell your car, being honest with the buyer are important.

d. If you want to selling your car, to be honest with the buyer is important.

19. Choose the best revision of the sentence.

Although today the boy was nice to my brother, they usually was quite mean to him.

a. Although today the boy was nice to my brother, they were usually quite mean to him.

b. Although today the boy was nice to my brother, he was usually quite mean to him.

c. Although today the boy were nice to my brother, he is usually quite mean to him.

d. Although today the boy was nice to my brother, he were usually quite mean to him.

20. Choose the sentence with the correct grammar.

a. The mother would not of punished her daughter if she could have avoided it.

b. The mother would not have punished her daughter if she could of avoided it.

c. The mother would not of punished her daughter if she could of avoided it.

d. The mother would not have punished her daughter if she could have avoided it.

21. Choose the sentence with the correct grammar.

a. There was scarcely no food in the pantry, because nobody ate at home.

b. There was scarcely any food in the pantry, because nobody ate at home.

c. There was scarcely any food in the pantry, because not nobody ate at home.

d. There was scarcely no food in the pantry, because not nobody ate at home.

22. Choose the sentence with the correct grammar.

a. Neither of them came with their bicycle.

b. Neither of them came with his bicycle.

c. Neither of them came with our bicycle.

d. None of the above.

23. Choose the sentence with the proper usage.

a. In spite of the bad weather yesterday, he can still attend the party.

b. In spite of the bad weather yesterday, he could still attend the party.

c. In spite of the bad weather yesterday, he may still attend the party.

d. None of the above.

24. Choose the sentence with the correct grammar.

a. Michael has lived in that house for forty years, while I has owned this one for only six weeks.

b. Michael have lived in that house for forty years, while I have owned this one for only six weeks.

c. Michael have lived in that house for forty years, while I has owned this one for only six weeks.

d. Michael has lived in that house for forty years, while I have owned this one for only six weeks.

25. Choose the sentence with the correct grammar.

a. The members of the team were asked to discuss with each other.

b. The members of the team were asked to discuss with one another.

c. Both of the above.

26. Choose the sentence with the proper usage.

a. The man raise up quickly.

b. The man rise up quickly.

c. The man rose up quickly.

d. None of the above.

27. Choose the sentence with the correct grammar.

a. He should have went to the appointment; instead, he went to the beach.

b. He should have gone to the appointment; instead, he went to the beach.

c. He should have went to the appointment; instead, he gone to the beach.

d. He should have gone to the appointment; instead, he gone to the beach.

28. Choose the sentence with the proper usage.

a. Their wages will be rised.

b. Their wages will be rose.

c. Their salaries will be raised.

d. None of the above.

30. Choose the sentence with the correct grammar.

a. Every doctor must come with his stethoscope

b. Every doctor must come with their stethoscope

c. Every doctor must come with our stethoscope

d. None of the above.

31. Choose the sentence with the correct grammar.

a. Lee pronounced it's name incorrectly; it's an impatiens, not an impatience.

b. Lee pronounced its name incorrectly; its an impatiens, not an impatience.

c. Lee pronounced it's name incorrectly; its an impatiens, not an impatience.

d. Lee pronounced its name incorrectly; it's an impatiens, not an impatience.

32. Choose the sentence with the proper usage.

a. She was nodding her head, her hips are swaying.

b. She was nodding her head, her hips is swaying.

c. She was nodding her head, her hips were swaying.

d. None of the above.

33. Choose the sentence with the correct usage.

a. They're going to graduate in June; after that, their best option will be to go there.

b. There going to graduate in June; after that, their best option will be to go there.

c. They're going to graduate in June; after that, there best option will be to go their.

d. Their going to graduate in June; after that, their best option will be to go there

34. Choose the sentence with the proper usage.

a. I shall arrive early and I will have breakfast with you.

b. I shall arrive early and I would have breakfast with you.

c. I shall arrive early and have breakfast with you.

d. None of the above.

35. Choose the sentence with the proper usage.

    a. The tables were laid by the students.

    b. The tables were lay by the students

    c. The tables were lie by the students

36. Choose the sentence with the correct usage.

    a. You're mistaken; that is not you're book.

    b. Your mistaken; that is not your book.

    c. You're mistaken; that is not your book.

    d. Your mistaken; that is not you're book.

37. Choose the sentence with the correct grammar.

    a. The teacher asked everybody is to submit his assignment by 9 a.m.

    b. The teacher asked everybody is to submit our assignment by 9 a.m.

    c. The teacher asked everybody is to submit their assignment by 9 a.m.

    d. None of the above.

38. Choose the sentence with the correct usage.

    a. He did not have to loose the race; if only his shoes weren't so lose!

    b. He did not have to lose the race; if only his shoes weren't so loose!

    c. He did not have to lose the race; if only his shoes weren't so lose!

    d. He did not have to loose the race; if only his shoes weren't so loose!

39. Choose the sentence with the correct usage.

a. The attorney did not want to prosecute the defendant; his goal was to prosecute the guilty party.

b. The attorney did not want to persecute the defendant; his goal was to persecute the guilty party.

c. The attorney did not want to prosecute the defendant; his goal was to persecute the guilty party.

d. The attorney did not want to persecute the defendant; his goal was to prosecute the guilty party.

40. Choose the sentence with the correct usage.

a. The speeches must precede the election; the election cannot proceed without hearing from the candidates.

b. The speeches must precede the election; the election cannot precede without hearing from the candidates.

c. The speeches must proceed the election; the election cannot precede without hearing from the candidates.

d. The speeches must proceed the election; the election cannot proceed without hearing from the candidates.

41. Choose the sentence with the correct usage.

a. Before a lawyer can rise an objection, he must first rise to his feet.

b. Before a lawyer can raise an objection, he must first raise to his feet.

c. Before a lawyer can raise an objection, he must first rise to his feet.

d. Before a lawyer can rise an objection, he must first raise to his feet.

42. Fill in the blank to make a correct sentence.

Neither of the Wright Brothers _____ that they would be successful with their flying machine.

    a. have any doubts

    b. has any doubts

    c. had any doubts

    d. will have any doubts

43. The weatherman on Channel 6 said that this has been the

    a. most hottest summer on record.

    b. most hottest summer on record.

    c. hottest summer on record.

    d. hotter summer on record.

44. Select the correct version of the sentence.

He is a cowered person.

    a. He is a cowardest person.

    b. He is a cowardly person.

    c. He is a coward person.

    d. The sentence is correct.

45. Select the correct version of the sentence.

Why did Mr. Simpson deny to help you?

    a. Why did Mr. Simpson refuse to help you?

    b. Why did Mr. Simpson resist to help you?

    c. Why did Mr. Simpson not accept to help you?

    d. The sentence is correct.

46. Select the correct version of the sentence.

She is the most cleverest girl in the class.

    a. She is the most clever girl in the class.

    b. She is the cleverest girl in the class.

    c. She is the most cleverer girl in the class.

    d. The sentence is correct.

47. Select the correct version of the sentence.

He lived in California since 1995.

    a. He had lived in California since 1995.

    b. He has been living in California since 1995.

    c. He has living in California since 1995.

    d. The sentence is correct.

48. Select the correct version of the sentence.

Please excuse me being late.

    a. Please excuse me for late.

    b. Please excuse my being late.

    c. Please excuse my being lateness.

    d. The sentence is correct.

49. Choose the sentence with the correct grammar.

    a. He doesn't have any money to buy clothes, and neither do I.

    b. He doesn't have any money to buy clothes, and neither does I.

    c. He don't have any money to buy clothes, and neither do I.

    d. He don't have any money to buy clothes, and neither does I.

50. Choose the sentence with the correct grammar.

   a. Because it really don't matter, I don't care if I go there.

   b. Because it really doesn't matter, I doesn't care if I go there.

   c. Because it really doesn't matter, I don't care if I go there.

   d. Because it really don't matter, I don't care if I go there.

Section IV – Vocabulary

1. Choose the adjective that means shocking, terrible or wicked.

   a. Pleasantries

   b. Heinous

   c. Shrewd

   d. Provencal

2. Choose the noun that means a person or thing that tells or announces the coming of someone or something.

   a. Harbinger

   b. Evasion

   c. Bleak

   d. Craven

3. Choose a word that means the same as the underlined word.

He wasn't especially generous. All the servings were very judicious.

   a. Abundant

   b. Careful

   c. Extravagant

   d. Careless

4. Fill in the blank.

Because of the growing use of _____ as a fuel, corn production has greatly increased.

    a. Alcohol

    b. Ethanol

    c. Natural gas

    d. Oil

5. Fill in the blank.

In heavily industrialized areas, the pollution of the air causes many to develop _____ diseases.

    a. Respiratory

    b. Cardiac

    c. Alimentary

    d. Circulatory

6. Choose the best definition of inherent.

    a. To receive money in a will

    b. An essential part of

    c. To receive money from a will

    d. None of the above

7. Choose the best definition of vapid.

    a. adj. tasteless or bland

    b. v. To inflict, as a revenge or punishment

    c. v. to convert into gas

    d. v. to go up in smoke

8. Choose the best definition of waif.

    a. n. a sick and hungry child

    b. n. an orphan staying in a foster home

    c. n. homeless child or stray

    d. n. a type of French bread eaten with cheese

9. Choose the adjective that means similar or identical.

a. Soluble

b. Assembly

c. Conclave

d. Homologous

10. Choose a word with the same meaning as the underlined word.

We used that operating system 20 years ago, now it is <u>obsolete</u>.

a. Functional

b. Disused

c. Obese

d. None of the Above

11. Choose the word with the same meaning as the underlined word

His bad manners really <u>rankle</u> me.

a. Annoy

b. Obsolete

c. Enliven

d. None of the above

12. Fill in the blank.

Because hydroelectric power is a _____ source of energy, its use is excellent for the environment.

a. Significant

b. Disposable

c. Renewable

d. Reusable

13. Choose the best definition of torpid.

    a. Fast
    b. Rapid
    c. Sluggish
    d. Violent

14. Choose the best definition of gregarious.

    a. Sociable
    b. Introverted
    c. Large
    d. Solitary

15. Choose the best definition of mutation.

    a. v. To utter with a loud and vehement voice
    b. n. change or alteration
    c. n. An act or exercise of will
    d. v. To cause to be one

16. Choose the best definition of lithe.

    a. adj. small in size
    b. adj. Artificial
    c. adj. flexible or plaint
    d. adj. fake

17. Choose the best definition of resent.

    a. adj. To express displeasure or indignation
    b. v. To cause to be one
    c. adj. Clumsy
    d. adj. strong feelings of love

18. Choose the adjective that means irrelevant not having substance or matter.

    a. Immaterial

    b. Prohibition

    c. Prediction

    d. Brokerage

19. Choose the adjective that means perfect, no faults or errors.

    a. Impeccable

    b. Formidable

    c. Genteel

    d. Disputation

20. Choose the best definition of pudgy.

    a. v. to draw general inferences

    b. Adj. fat, plump and overweight

    c. n. permanence

    d. adj. spoilt or bad condition

21. Choose the best definition of alloy.

    a. To mix with something superior

    b. To mix

    c. To mix with something inferior

    d. To purify

22. Fill in the blank.

The process required the use of highly _____ liquids, so fire extinguishers were everywhere in the factory.

   a. Erratic

   b. Combustible

   c. Stable

   d. Neutral

23. Choose the best definition for the underlined word.

We don't want to hear the whole thing. Just the <u>salient</u> facts please.

   a. Irrelevant

   b. Erroneous

   c. Relevant

   d. Trivial

24. Choose the best definition for the underlined word.

I don't know why he is being so nice. I am sure he has an <u>ulterior</u> motive.

   a. Inferior

   b. Additional

   c. Simplistic

   d. Unfortunate

25. Choose the noun that means ruling council of a military government.

   a. Retribution

   b. Counsel

   c. Virago

   d. Junta

26. Choose a noun that means someone who takes more time than necessary.

    a. Manager

    b. Haggard

    c. Laggard

    d. Expound

27. Choose an adjective that means lacking enthusiasm, strength or energy.

    a. Hapless

    b. Languid

    c. Ubiquitous

    d. Promiscuous

28. Choose a word that means the same as the underlined word.

I still don't know exactly. That isn't <u>conclusive</u> evidence.

    a. Undeterred

    b. Unrelenting

    c. Unfortunate

    d. Definitive

29. Choose the best definition of mollify.

    a. To anger

    b. To modify

    c. To irritate

    d. To soothe

30. Choose the best definition of redundant.

    a. Backup

    b. Necessary repetition

    c. Unnecessary repetition

    d. No repetition

31. Choose the best definition of raucous.

    a. Adj. Pedantic; academic; for teaching

    b. Adj. contemptuous, scornful

    c. adj. Not essential under the circumstances

    d. adj. harsh or rough sounding

32. Choose the noun that means a person of influence, rank or distinction.

    a. Consummate

    b. Sinister

    c. Accolade

    d. Magnate

33. Choose the word that means the same as the underlined word.

The warehouse went bankrupt so all of the furniture has to be <u>sold.</u>

    a. Dissected

    b. Liquidated

    c. Destroyed

    d. Bought

34. Choose the word that means the same as the underlined word.

He sold the property when he didn't even own it. The whole thing was a <u>fraud</u>.

    a. Hoax

    b. Feign

    c. Defile

    d. Default

35. Choose the best definition of bicker.

    a. Chat

    b. Discuss

    c. Argue

    d. Debate

36. Choose a noun that means a lingering disease or ailment of the human body.

    a. Treatment

    b. Frontal

    c. Malady

    d. Assiduous

37. Choose the word that means the same as the underlined word.

Just because she is supervisor, doesn't mean we have to <u>cower</u> in front of her.

    a. Foible

    b. Grovel

    c. Humiliate

    d. Indispose

38. Choose the best definition of maverick.

    a. Rebel

    b. Conformist

    c. Unconventional

    d. Conventional

39. Choose the adjective that means relating to a wedding or marriage.

    a. Nefarious

    b. Fluctuate

    c. Nuptial

    d. Flatulence

40. Choose the adjective that means open display or apparent.

    a. Ostensible

    b. Sign-post

    c. Revealing

    d. Harrowing

41. Choose the word that means the same as the underlined word.
Her attitude was very <u>casual</u>.

    a. Idle

    b. Nonchalant

    c. Portly

    d. Portend

42. Choose the word that means the same as the underlined word.
The machine <u>powderizes</u> the rock.

    a. Quells

    b. Pulverizes

    c. Eradicates

    d. Segments

43. Choose the best definition of tenuous.

    a. Strong

    b. Tense

    c. Firm

    d. Weak

44. Choose the noun that means a sheet of paper that can be folded into 8 leaves.

    a. Octagon

    b. Harangue

    c. Octavo

    d. Wreckage

45. Choose the word that means the same as the underlined word.

The water in the pond has been sitting for so long it is <u>dead</u>.

    a. Stagnant

    b. Sediment

    c. Stupor

    d. Residue

46. Choose the word with the same meaning as the underlined word.

She didn't listen to a thing and <u>rejected</u> all the objections.

    a. Manipulated

    b. Mired

    c. Furtive

    d. Rebuffed

47. Choose the best definition of pandemonium.

    a. Chaos

    b. Orderly

    c. Quiet

    d. Noisy

48. Choose the best definition of perpetual.

    a. Continuous

    b. Slowly

    c. Over a very long time

    d. Motion

49. Choose the adjective that means appearing weak or pale.

    a. Pallid

    b. Palliative

    c. Deviant

    d. Expatiate

50. Choose the word that means the same as the underlined word.
He loaned me the money last month and is going to repay me tomorrow.

   a. Reimburse

   b. Reinstate

   c. Reconcile

   d. Rebuff

Section V – Science

1. A soccer ball is kicked and travels at a velocity of 12 m/sec. After 60 seconds, it comes to a stop. What is the acceleration?

   a. -0.2 m/sec^2

   b. 0.2 m/sec^2

   c. 1 m/sec^2

   d. 0.5 m/sec^2

2. A molecule of water contains hydrogen and oxygen in a 1:8 ratio by mass. This is a statement of

   a. The law of multiple proportions

   b. The law of conservation of mass

   c. The law of conservation of energy

   d. The law of constant composition

3. Electrons play a critical role in

   a. Electricity

   b. Magnetism

   c. Thermal conductivity

   d. All of the above

4. An idea concerning a phenomena and possible explanations for that phenomena is a/an

    a. Theory.

    b. Experiment.

    c. Inference.

    d. Hypothesis.

5. Define chromosomes.

    a. Structures in a cell nucleus that carry genetic material.

    b. Consist of thousands of DNA strands.

    c. Total 46 in a normal human cell.

    d. All of the above

6. A base is

    a. A compound that reacts with an acid to form a salt.

    b. A molecule or ion that captures hydrogen ions.

    c. A molecule or ion that donates an electron pair to form a chemical bond.

    d. All of the above are true

7. Which disease of the circulatory system is one of the most frequent causes of death in North America?

    a. The cold

    b. Pneumonia

    c. Arthritis

    d. Heart disease

8. How fast is a person walking if they travel 1000 meters in 20 minutes?

    a. 25 meters/minute

    b. 50 meters/minute

    c. 100 meters/minute

    d. None of the above

9. A substance containing atoms of more than one element in a definite ratio is called a(n)

a. Compound.

b. Element.

c. Mixture.

d. Molecule.

10. Which of the following describes a plasma membrane?

a. Lipids with embedded proteins

b. An outer lipid layer and an inner lipid layer

c. Proteins embedded in lipid bilayer

d. Altering protein and lipid layers

11. Protein biosynthesis is defined as

a. The addition of protein to foods that lack it.

b. Ribosomes synthesizing proteins in the endoplasmic reticulum.

c. The process of proteasomes degrading cytoplasm.

d. Proteins "flowing" through the ER into the plasma membrane.

12. When we speak of separating organelles through centrifugation, we're speaking of

a. Cell fractionation

b. Flow cytometry

c. Immunoprecipation

d. Detergents

13. What is the difference between Strong Nuclear Force and Weak Nuclear Force?

a. The Strong Nuclear Force is an attractive force that binds protons and neutrons and maintains the structure of the nucleus, and the Weak Nuclear Force is responsible for the radioactive beta decay and other subatomic reactions.

b. The Strong Nuclear Force is responsible for the radioactive beta decay and other subatomic reactions, and the Weak Nuclear Force is an attractive force that binds protons and neutrons and maintains the structure of the nucleus.

c. The Weak Nuclear Force is feeble and the Strong Nuclear Force is robust.

d. The Strong Nuclear Force is a negative force that releases protons and neutrons and threatens the structure of the nucleus, and the Weak Nuclear Force is an attractive force that binds protons and neutrons and maintains the structure of the nucleus.

14. 1000 N force is applied to a concrete block that weights 500 pounds. How fast will this force accelerate the block?

a. 1 m/sec²

b. 2 m/sec²

c. 3 m/sec²

d. 5 m/sec²

15. What type of research deals with the quality, type or components of a group, substance, or mixture?

a. Quantitative

b. Dependent

c. Scientific

d. Qualitative

16. When a measurement is recorded, it includes the _____ _____, **which are all the digits that are certain plus one uncertain digit.**

    a. Major figures
    b. Significant figures
    c. Relative figures
    d. Relevant figures

17. The equation E = mc² is based on the _____, **and states that** _____ **equals** _____ **times the** _____²**.**

    a. The equation $E = mc^2$ is based on the 2nd Law of Thermodynamics, and states that Mass equals Energy times (the Velocity of light)².

    b. The equation $E = mc^2$ is based on the Law of Conservation of Mass and Energy, and states that Energy equals Mass times (the Velocity of light)².

    c. The equation $E = mc^2$ is based on the 1st Law of Thermodynamics, and states that Mass equals Energy times (the Velocity of sound)².

    d. The equation $E = mc^2$ is based on the Law of Conservation of Mass and Energy, and states that the Velocity of light equals Energy times (the Mass)².

18. Describe a pH indicator.

    a. A pH indicator measures hydrogen ions in a solution and show pH on a color scale.

    b. A pH indicator measures oxygen ions in a solution and show pH on a color scale.

    c. A pH indicator many different types of ions in a solution and shows pH on a color scale.

    d. None of the above.

19. All acids turn blue litmus paper

a. Blue

b. Red

c. Green

d. White

20. What type of bonds involve a complete sharing of electrons and occurs most commonly between atoms that have partially filled outer shells or energy levels?

a. Covalent

b. Ionic

c. Hydrogen

d. Proportional

21. What can accept a hydrogen ion and can react with fats to form soaps?

a. Acid

b. Salt

c. Base

d. Foundation

22. Which, if any, of the following statements are true?

a. Water boils at approximately 100 °C (212 °F) at standard atmospheric pressure.

b. The boiling point is the temperature at which the vapor pressure is higher than the atmospheric pressure around the water.

c. Water boils at a higher temperature in areas of lower pressure.

d. All of the above statements are true.

23. Which gene, whose presence as a single copy, controls the expression of a trait?

 a. Principal gene

 b. Latent gene

 c. Recessive gene

 d. Dominant gene

24. What is the mathematical function that gives the amplitude of a wave as a function of position (and sometimes, as a function of time and/or electron spin)?

 a. Wavelength

 b. Frequency

 c. Wavenumber

 d. Wavefunction

25. Which of the following is not a habitat where bacteria commonly grow?

 a. Soil

 b. The vacuum of space

 c. Radioactive waste

 d. Deep in the earth's crust

26. Within taxonomy, plants and animals are considered two basic

 a. Families

 b. Kingdoms

 c. Domains

 d. Genus

27. Most of the elements on the periodic table can be classified as

    a. Nonmetals

    b. Metals

    c. Metalloids

    d. Gas

28. What is a chemical involved in, but not changed by, a chemical reaction by which chemical bonds are weakened and reactions accelerated.

    a. A propellant

    b. A reagent

    c. A catalyst

    d. None of the above

29. Organisms grouped into the _____ Kingdom include all unicellular organisms lacking a definite cellular arrangement such as _____ and _____.

    a. Fungi, bacteria, algae

    b. Protista, bacteria, amphibian

    c. Protista, bacteria, algae

    d. Plantae, bacteria, algae

30. Which of these statements about metals are true?

    a. A metal is a substance that conducts heat and electricity.

    b. A metal is shiny and reflects many colors of light, and can be hammered into sheets or drawn into wire.

    c. All of these statements are true.

    d. About 80% of the known chemical elements are metals.

31. What type of bond does a reaction of elements with low electronegativity (almost empty outer shells) with elements with high electronegativity (mostly full outer shells) create?

    a. Hydrogen

    b. Covalent

    c. Ionic

    d. Nuclear

32. Which of the following is not an infectious bacterial disease?

    a. Cholera

    b. Anthrax

    c. Leprosy

    d. AIDS

33. Define a biological class.

    a. A collection of similar or like living entities.

    b. Two or more animals in a group, all having the same parent.

    c. All animals sharing the same living environment.

    d. All plant life that share the same physical properties.

34. Which, if any, of the following statements about prokaryotic cells is false?

    a. Prokaryotic cells include such organisms as E. coli and Streptococcus.

    b. Prokaryotic cells lack internal membranes and organelles.

    c. Prokaryotic cells break down food using cellular respiration and fermentation.

    d. All of these statements are true.

35. 1000 N force is applied to a concrete block that weights 500 pounds. How fast will this force accelerate the block?

    a. -2 m/sec^2

    b. 2 m/sec^2

    c. 4 m/sec^2

    d. 5 m/sec^2

36. What is the process of converting observed phenomena into data called?

    a. Calculation

    b. Measurement

    c. Valuation

    d. Estimation

37. What law states that when two elements combine to form more than one compound, the weight of one element that combines with a fixed weight of the other are in a ratio of small whole numbers?

    a. The Law of Multiple Proportions

    b. The Law of Definite Proportions

    c. The Law of the Conservation of Energy

    d. The Law of Averages

38. What word describes the wide diversity of sizes and shapes found in bacteria?

    a. Morphologies

    b. Cosmologies

    c. Proteins

    d. Spirilla

39. The mass number of an atom is

    a. The total number of particles that make it up.

    b. The total weight of an atom.

    c. The total mass of an atom.

    d. None of the above.

40. Which of these statements about mechanical energy is/are true?

a. Mechanical energy is the energy that is possessed by an object due to its motion or due to its position.

b. Mechanical energy can be either kinetic energy (energy of motion) or potential energy (stored energy of position).

c. Objects have mechanical energy if they are in motion.

d. All of the above.

41. What three processes are involved in cell division of Eukaryotic cells?

a. Meiosis, mitosis, and interphase

b. Meiosis, mitosis, and interphase

c. Mitosis, kinematisis, and interphase

d. Mitosis, cytokinesis, and interphase

42. The _____ _____ of an element equals the number of protons in an atomic nucleus, and, along with the element symbol is one of two alternate ways to label an element.

a. Atomic unit

b. Atomic number

c. Atomic orbital

d. Nuclear number

43. Which of the following statements, if any, are correct?

a. pH is a measure of effective concentration of hydrogen ions in a solution, and is approximately related to the molarity of H+ by pH = - log [H+]

b. pH is a measure of effective concentration of oxygen ions in a solution, and is approximately related to the molarity of O+ by pH = - log [O+]

c. pH is a measure of effective concentration of hydrogen atoms in a solution, and is approximately related to the polarity of H+ by pH = - log [H+]

d. Acidity is a measure of effective concentration of hydrogen ions in a solution, and is approximately related to the molarity of H+ by pH = - log [H+]

44. What chain of nucleotides plays an important role in the creation of new proteins?

a. Deoxyribonucleic acid (DNA) is a chain of nucleotides that plays an important role in the creation of new proteins.

b. Ribonucleic acid (RNA) is a chain of nucleotides that plays an important role in the creation of new proteins.

c. There are no chains of nucleotides that play a role in the creation of proteins.

d. None of the above.

45. How much force is needed to accelerate a car that weights 200 kg to 5 m/s²?

a. 40 N

b. 200 N

c. 1000 N

d. 1500 N

46. What law states that every chemical compound contains fixed and constant proportions (by weight) of its constituent elements?

    a. The Law of Multiple Proportions

    b. The Law of the Preservation of Matter

    c. The Law of the Conservation of Energy

    d. The Law of Definite Proportions

47. Four factors that affect rates of reaction are

    a. Barometric pressure, particle size, concentration, and the presence of a facilitator.

    b. Temperature, particle size, concentration, and the presence of a catalyst.

    c. Temperature, container material, elevation, and the presence of instability.

    d. Volatility, particle size, concentration, and the presence of a catalyst.

48. What is the term used for bacterial species which are spherical in shape?

    a. Bacilli

    b. Spirilla

    c. Cocci

    d. Spirochaetes

49. A practical test designed with the intention that its results will be relevant to a particular theory or set of theories is a/an _____.

    a. Experiment

    b. Practicum

    c. Theory

    d. Design

50. If 3 moles of sugar is dissolved to form 2 liters of a solution, calculate the molarity of the solution.

   a. 1 M solution

   b. 1.5 M solution

   c. 2 M solution

   d. 2.5 M solution

51. Electricity is a general term encompassing a variety of phenomena resulting from the presence and flow of electric charge. Which of the following statements about electricity is/are true?

   a. Electrically charged matter is influenced by, and produces, electromagnetic fields.

   b. Electric current is a movement or flow of electrically charged particles.

   c. Electric potential is a fundamental interaction between the magnetic field and the presence and motion of an electric charge.

   d. All of the statements are true.

52. Strong chemical bonds include

   a. Dipole - dipole interactions

   b. Hydrogen bonding

   c. Covalent or ionic bonds

   d. None of the above

53. A javelin is thrown into a field at 18 m/s. if the Javelin weighs 1.5 kg, what is the momentum?

   a. 1.2 kg x m/s into the field

   b. 12 kg x m/s into the field

   c. 27 kg x m/s into the field

   d. 2.7 kg x m/s into the field

54. Which of these object has greater momentum, a 2 kg truck moving east at 3.5 m/s or a 4.3 kg truck moving south at 1.5 m/s?

a. The first truck at 7 kg x m/s moving east

b. The second truck at 7.45 kg x m/s due south

c. The first truck at 6.45 kg x m/s due east

d. The second truck at 7 kg x m/s due south

55. What is the measure of an experiment's ability to yield the same or compatible results in different clinical experiments or statistical trials?

a. Variability

b. Validity

c. Control measure

d. Reliability

56. Genes control heredity in man and other organisms. This gene is

a. a segment of RNA or DNA.

b. a bead like structure on the chromosomes.

c. a protein molecule.

d. a segment of RNA.

57. One factor that affects rates of reaction is concentration. Which of these statements about concentration is/are correct?

a. A higher concentration of reactants causes more effective collisions per unit time, leading to an increased reaction rate.

b. A lower concentration of reactants causes more effective collisions per unit time, leading to an increased reaction rate.

c. A higher concentration of reactants causes more effective collisions per unit time, leading to a decreased reaction rate.

d. A higher concentration of reactants causes less effective collisions per unit time, leading to an increased reaction rate.

58. Describe each chemical element in the periodic table.

a. Each chemical element has a unique atomic number representing the number of electrons in its nucleus.

b. Each chemical element has a varying atomic number depending on the number of protons in its nucleus.

c. Each chemical element has a unique atomic number representing the number of protons in its nucleus.

d. None of the above.

59. Which of the following statements about nonmetals are true?

a. A nonmetal is a substance that conducts heat and electricity poorly.

b. The majority of the known chemical elements are nonmetals.

c. A nonmetal is brittle or waxy or gaseous.

d. All of the statements are true.

60. The molarity of 5 liters of a salt solution is 0.5 M of salt solution. Calculate the moles of salt in the solution.

a. 2 Moles

b. 2.5 Moles

c. 2.75 Moles

d. 3 Moles

61. A solution with a pH value of less than 7 is

a. Acid solution

b. Base solution

c. Neutral pH solution

d. None of the above

62. What is the distance between adjacent peaks (or adjacent troughs) on a wave?

    a. Frequency

    b. Wavenumber

    c. Wave oscillation

    d. Wavelength

63. An object that weighs 500 g is rolling along the road at 3.5 m/s. What is the momentum of the object?

    a. 124.9 kg x m/s along road

    b. 17. 50 kg x m/s along road

    c. 1750 kg x m/s along road

    d. 1.75 kg x m/s along road

64. Is a catalyst changed by a reaction?

    a. Yes

    b. No

    c. It may be changed depending on the other chemicals

65. The _____ is the prediction that an observed difference is due to chance alone and not due to a systematic cause; this hypothesis is tested by statistical analysis, and either accepted or rejected.

    a. Null hypothesis

    b. Hypothesis

    c. Control

    d. Variable

66. In science, industry, and statistics, the _____ of a measurement system is the degree of closeness of measurements of a quantity to its actual (true) value.

    a. Mistake

    b. Uncertainty

    c. Accuracy

    d. Error

67. The horizontal rows of the periodic table are known as

    a. Groups

    b. Periods

    c. Series

    d. Columns

68. Which, if any, of these statements about solubility are correct?

    a. The solubility of a substance is its concentration in a saturated solution.

    b. Substances with solubilities much less than 1 g/100 mL of solvent are usually considered insoluble.

    c. A saturated solution is one which does not dissolve any more solute.

    d. All of these statements are correct.

69. Describe a valence shell.

    a. Is the shell corresponding to the highest value of principal quantum number in the atom.

    b. The valence electrons in this shell are on average closer to the nucleus than other electrons.

    c. They are rarely directly involved in chemical reaction.

    d. None of the above are true.

70. To calculate the molarity of a solution when the solute is given in grams and the volume of the solution is given in milliliters, you must first

a. Convert grams to moles, but leave the volume of solution in milliliters.

b. Convert volume of solution in milliliters to liters, but leave grams to moles.

c. Convert grams to moles, and convert volume of solution in milliliters to liters.

d. None of the above.

71. What is the atomic number for Hydrogen?

a. 11

b. 2

c. 1

d. 5

72. The vertical columns of the periodic table are known as

a. Series

b. Groups

c. Periods

d. Columns

73. The ____ of a distribution is the difference between the maximum value and the minimum value.

a. Distribution

b. Range

c. Mode

d. Median

74. A cannon ball weighing 35 kg is shot from a cannon towards the east at 220m/s, calculate the momentum of the cannon ball.

  a. 7500 kg m/s east

  b. 7700 kg m/s east

  c. 8000 kg m/s east

  d. 8500 kg m/s east

75. Which, if any, of the following statements describing acids are correct?

  a. An acid is a compound containing detachable hydrogen ions.

  b. An acid is a compound that can accept a pair of electrons from a base.

  c. A and B are correct

  d. None of the above

Section VI - Anatomy and Physiology

1. The stomach and colon are both in the

  a. Left Upper Quadrant.

  b. Right Upper Quadrant.

  c. Right Lower Quadrant.

  d. Left Lower Quadrant.

2. The stomach is located in

  a. LLQ.

  b. LUQ.

  c. RUQ.

  d. RLQ.

3. An example of something that increases a person's metabolism is

    a. Aerobic exercise.

    b. Mental exercise.

    c. Eating a fatty diet.

    d. Reading.

4. Nerve tissue is made up of cells known as

    a. Neurons.

    b. Protons.

    c. Molecules.

    d. Atoms.

5. Which sub-layer of skin gives it flexibility?

    a. The dermis

    b. Epidermis

    c. Subdermis

    d. Dermatology

6. What makes it sometimes difficult to diagnose an ailment within the musculoskeletal system?

    a. Bones resist X-rays.

    b. There are no diseases associated with the musculo-skeletal system.

    c. Its close proximity to other organs within the body.

    d. Its distant proximity away from other organs within the body.

7. One disease of the circulatory system which is often mistakenly thought to be a heart attack is

    a. Cardiac arrest.

    b. High blood pressure.

    c. Angina.

    d. Acid reflux.

8. An example of an important side-benefit of the respiratory system is

a. The air allows whistling.

b. The oxygen expelled can be recycled for other uses.

c. The air being expelled from the mouth allows for speaking.

d. The air expelled from the body also expels disease and germs.

9. The process by which the immune system adapts over time to be more efficient in recognizing pathogens is known as

a. Acquired immunity.

b. AIDS.

c. Pathogens.

d. Acquired deficiency.

10. A common digestive affliction that most people suffer at one time or other is

a. Stomach cancer.

b. Ulceritis.

c. Indigestion.

d. The flu.

11. One example of the blood stream's part in the digestive system is

a. Preventing infection.

b. Carrying urea to the kidneys.

c. Expelling the urea from the body.

d. The blood stream has no part in the digestive system.

12. The intestines are located in

a. LUQ.

b. LLQ.

c. RLQ.

d. All of the above.

13. Fluid balance is important, because the human body loses water every day through urination, perspiration, feces, and

a. Breathing.

b. Resting.

c. Meditating.

d. Outbursts of temper.

14. The three layers of skin are

a. Proton, neuron and nucleus.

b. Epidural, Mitochondria and chromosome

c. Inner, outer and local.

d. Epidermis, dermis and sub dermis.

15. An example of a minor ailment of the integumentary system is

a. Skin cancer.

b. Acne.

c. Common cold.

d. Flu.

16. What is osteoporosis?

a. A brain disorder that moves to the leg bones.

b. A condition in which nerves become fragile.

c. An ailment in which muscles deteriorate.

d. An ailment in which bones become fragile because of loss of tissue.

17. What is a more common name for the circulatory system disease known as hypertension?

a. Anemia

b. High blood pressure

c. Angina

d. Cardiac arrest

18. An example of a disease of the lungs that is caused or made worse by smoking is

a. Emphysema.

b. Strep throat.

c. Muscular dystrophy.

d. Leukemia.

19. Which cells are an important weapon in the fight against infection?

a. Red blood cells

b. White blood cells

c. Barrier cells

d. Virus cells

20. Besides the kidney, the other major organ that takes part in the body's urinary system is

a. The penis

b. The Liver

c. The Stomach

d. The Bladder

21. Which of these describes the bladder?

a. A pea-sized, circular organ.

b. A balloon shaped, muscular organ.

c. A squarish organ about the size of the small intestine.

d. A triangular organ the same size as the heart.

22. An example of appendages contained within the integumentary system are

    a. Lungs

    b. Hair and nails

    c. Nostrils

    d. Ears

23. What is an example of a serious ailment of the integumentary system?

    a. Acne

    b. Skin cancer

    c. Heart disease

    d. High blood pressure

24. What is a condition in which the heart beats too fast, too slow, or with an irregular beat is called?

    a. Hypertension

    b. Angina

    c. Cardiac arrest

    d. Arrythmia

25. What is an example of an early response by the immune system to infection?

    a. Inhalation

    b. Inflammation

    c. Respiration

    d. Exhalation

Answer Key

1. B

We can infer an important part of the respiratory system are the lungs. From the passage, "Molecules of oxygen and carbon dioxide are passively exchanged, by diffusion, between the gaseous external environment and the blood. This exchange process occurs in the alveolar region of the lungs."

Therefore, one of the primary functions for the respiratory system is the exchange of oxygen and carbon dioxide, and this process occurs in the lungs. We can therefore infer that the lungs are an important part of the respiratory system.

2. C

The process by which molecules of oxygen and carbon dioxide are passively exchanged is diffusion.

This is a definition type question. Scan the passage for references to "oxygen," "carbon dioxide," or "exchanged."

3. A

The organ that plays an important role in gas exchange in amphibians is the skin.

Scan the passage for references to "amphibians," and find the answer.

4. A

The three physiological zones of the respiratory system are Conducting, transitional, respiratory zones.

5. B

This warranty does not cover a product that you have tried to fix yourself. From paragraph two, "This limited warranty does not cover ... any unauthorized disassembly, repair, or modification. "

6. C

ABC Electric could either replace or repair the fan, provided the other conditions are met. ABC Electric has the option to repair or replace.

7. B

The warranty does not cover a stove damaged in a flood. From the passage, "This limited warranty does not cover any damage to the product from improper installation, accident, abuse, misuse, natural disaster, insufficient or excessive electrical supply, abnormal mechanical or environmental conditions."

A flood is an "abnormal environmental condition," and a natural disaster, so it is not covered.

8. A

A missing part is an example of defective workmanship. This is an error made in the manufacturing process. A defective part is not considered workmanship.

9. B

The first paragraph tells us that myths are a true account of the remote past.

The second paragraph tells us that, "myths generally take place during a primordial age, when the world was still young, before achieving its current form."

Putting these two together, we can infer that humankind used myth to explain how the world was created.

10. A

This passage is about different types of stories. First, the passage explains myths, and then compares other types of stories to myths.

11. B

From the passage, "Unlike myths, folktales can take place at any time and any place, and the natives do not usually consider them true or sacred."

12. B

This question gives options with choices for the three different characteristics of myth and legend. The options are,

- True or not true

- Takes place in modern day

- About ordinary people

For this type of question, where two things are compared for different characteristics, you can easily eliminate wrong answers using only one choice. Take myths: myths are believed to be true, do not take place in modern day, and are not about ordinary people.

Make a list as follows,

- True or not true - True

- Takes place in modern day - No

- About ordinary people - No

Now check the options quickly. Option A is wrong (myths do not take place in modern day). Option B looks good. Put a check beside it. Option C is incorrect (myths are about ordinary people), and Option D is incorrect (myths are not true), so the answer must be Option B.

13. B
This passage describes the different categories for traditional stories. The other options are facts from the passage, not the main idea of the passage. The main idea of a passage will always be the most general statement. For example, Option A, Myths, fables, and folktales are not the same thing, and each describes a specific type of story. This is a true statement from the passage, but not the main idea of the passage, since the passage also talks about how some cultures may classify a story as a myth and others as a folktale.

The statement, from Option B, Traditional stories can be categorized in different ways by different people, is a more general statement that describes the passage.

14. B
Option B is the best choice, categories that group traditional stories according to certain characteristics.

Options A and C are false and can be eliminated right away. Option D is designed to confuse. Option D may be true, but it is not mentioned in the passage.

15. D
The best answer is D, traditional stories themselves are a part of the larger category of folklore, which may also include costumes, gestures, and music.

All of the other options are false. Traditional stories are part of the larger category of Folklore, which includes other things, not the other way around.

16. A
There is a distinct difference between a myth and a legend, both are folktales.

17. B
The techniques for controlling insects are taken directly from the first sentence.

18. B
The inference is humans control pests because they damage crops.

19. A
Feeding on crops is the best choice, even though A and C are also correct.

20. B
When someone is avid about something that means they are highly interested in the subject. The context clues are dull and boring, because they define the opposite of avid.

Option D is incorrect because you can be a fast reader and still not be interested in what you have read.

21. A
The author is using a simile to compare the books to medicine. Medicine is what you take when you want to feel better. They are suggesting that if a person wants to feel good, they should read Dr. Seuss' books.

Option B is incorrect because there is no mention of a doctor's office.
Option C is incorrect because it is using the literal meaning of medicine and the author is using medicine in a figurative way.

22. D

The publisher is described as intelligent because he knew to get in touch with a famous author to develop a book that children would be interested in reading.

Option A is incorrect because we can assume that all book publishers must know how to read.
Option D is incorrect because there is no mention in the article about how well The Cat in the Hat sold when it was first published.

23. B

The passage describes in detail how Dr. Seuss had a great effect on the lives of children through his writing. It names several of his books, tells how he helped children become avid readers and explains his style of writing.

Options A, C and D are incorrect because they refer to just one single fact about the passage.
Option B is correct because it encompasses ALL the facts in the passage, not just one single fact

24. D

This question is designed to confuse by presenting different options for the two chemicals, oxygen and carbon dioxide. One is produced, and one is reduced. Read the passage carefully to see which is reduced and which is produced.

25. B

The inference is botanists have not surveyed all the tropical areas so they do not know the number of species.

26. A

This is taken directly from the passage.

27. D

Tree-ferns survived the Carboniferous period. This is a fact-based question about the Carboniferous period. "Carboniferous" is an unusual word, so the fastest way to answer this question is to scan the pas-sage for the word "Carboniferous" and find the answer.

28. B

Here is the passage with the oldest to youngest trees.

The earliest trees were [1] tree ferns and horsetails, which grew in forests in the Carboniferous period. Tree ferns still survive, but the only surviving horsetails are no longer in tree form. Later, in the Triassic period, [2] conifers and ginkgos, appeared, [3] followed by flowering plants after that in the Cretaceous period.

29. B
The time limit for radar detectors is 14 days. Since you made the purchase 15 days ago, you do not qualify for the guarantee.

30. A
We know that an annex is like an attic because the text states the annex was above Otto Frank's building. Option B is incorrect because an office building doesn't have bedrooms.

31. B
The diary has been published in 55 languages so people all over the world can learn about Anne. That is why the passage says it has been continuously in print.
Option A is incorrect because it is too vague. Option C is incorrect because it was published after Anne died and she did not write in all three languages.
Option D is incorrect because the passage does not give us any information about what languages Otto Frank spoke.

32. C
You use process of elimination to figure this out. Option A cannot be the correct answer otherwise the passage would have simply said that Anne and Margot both died of starvation.
Options B and D cannot be correct because the Germans had done something specifically to murder Anne, the passage would have stated that directly.
By process of elimination, C has to be the correct answer.

33. D
We can figure this out using context clues. The paragraph is talking about Anne's diary and so, outlet in this instance is a place where Anne can pour her feelings.

Option A is incorrect. This is the literal meaning of the

word outlet and the passage is using the figurative meaning.

Option B is incorrect because that is the secondary literal meaning of the word outlet, as in an outlet mall. Again, we are looking for figurative meaning.

Option C is incorrect because there are no clues in the text to support it.

34. A

We can infer that an important purpose of the circulatory system is that of fighting diseases.

35. B

Humans have a closed circulatory system.

36. C

Besides blood, the heart and the blood vessels form the cardiovascular system.

37. B

The digestive system, along with the circulatory system, helps provide nutrients to keep the human heart pumping.

38. A

Helen's parents hired Anne to teach Helen to communicate.

Option B is incorrect because the passage states Anne had trouble finding her way around, which means she could walk.

39. B

The correct answer because that fact is stated directly in the passage. The passage explains that Anne taught Helen to hear by allowing her to feel the vibrations in her throat.

40. A

We can infer that Anne is a patient teacher because she did not leave or lose her temper when Helen bit or hit her; she just kept trying to teach Helen.

Option B is incorrect because Anne taught Helen to read and talk. Option C is incorrect because Anne could hear. She was partly blind, not deaf. Option D is incorrect because it does not have to do with patience.

41. B
The passage states that it was hard for anyone but Anne to understand Helen when she spoke.

Option A is incorrect because the passage does not mention Helen spoke a foreign language. Option C is incorrect because there is no mention of how quiet or loud Helen's voice was. Option D is incorrect because we know from reading the passage that Helen did learn to speak.

42. A
The main idea of this passage is that the human skeleton is an important and complicated system of the body.

We can infer the skeleton is important because it protects important organs like brain, lungs and heart. We know the skeleton is complicated because it consists of several parts, (ligaments, tendons, muscles and cartilage) and 206 bones.

This general statement best describes the passage. The other choices are details mentioned in the passage.

43. A
There are three bones are located in the human middle ear. This is a fact-based question taken directly from the passage.

44. B
The number of bones stays the same throughout one's lifetime is not true. From the passage, "There are 206 bones in the adult human skeleton, which varies between individuals and with age."

45. D
The appendicular skeleton attached to the axial skeleton. This is a fact-based question.

Section II – Math

1. D
8327 – 1278 = 7049

2. B
294 X 21 = 6174

3. C
1278 + 4920 = 6198

4. A
285 * 12 = 3420

5. C
4120 – 3216 = 904

6. D
2417 + 1004 = 3421
7. B
1440 ÷ 12 = 120

8. C
2713 – 1308 = 1405

9. D
$x^2 + 4x = 5$, $x^2 + 4x - 5 = 0$, $x^2 + 5x - x - 5 = 0$, factoring x(x + 5) - 1(x + 5) = 0, (x + 5)(x-1)=0. x + 5 = 0 or x - 1 = 0, x = 0 - 5 or x = 0 + 1, x = -5 or x = 1, either b or c.

10. C
Open parenthesis: 2a + 2b = 4ab, divide both sides by 2 = a + b = 2ab or a + b = ab + ab, therefore a = ab and b = ab, therefore a = b.

11. B
Let the XY represent the initial number, X + Y = 12, YX = XY+ 36, Only b = 48 satisfies both equations above from the given options.

12. B
Number of absent students = 83 – 72 = 11

Percentage of absent students is found by proportioning the number of absent students to total number of students in the class = $11 \cdot 100/83 = 13.25$

Checking the answers, we round 13.25 to the nearest whole number: 13%

13. B
Let the father's age=Y, and Kate's age=X, therefore Y=32+X, in 5 years y=5x, substituting for Y will be 5x = 32+X, 5x – x = 32, 4X=32, X= 32/8, x = 8, Kate will be 8 in 5 yrs time, so Kate's present age = 8 - 5 = 3.

14. A
This is a simple direct proportion problem:
If Lynn can type 1 page in p minutes,

    she can type x pages in 5 minutes

We do cross multiplication: $x \cdot p = 5 \cdot 1$

Then,

$x = 5/p$

15. A
This is an inverse ration problem.

$1/x = 1/a + 1/b$ where a is the time Sally can paint a house, b is the time John can paint a house, x is the time Sally and John can together paint a house.

So,

$1/x = 1/4 + 1/6$ ... We use the least common multiple in the denominator that is 24:

$1/x = 6/24 + 4/24$

$1/x = 10/24$

$x = 24/10$

$x = 2.4$ hours.

In other words; 2 hours + 0.4 hours = 2 hours + $0.4 \cdot 60$ minutes

= 2 hours 24 minutes

16. D
The cost of the dishwasher = $450

15% discount amount = 450•15/100 = $67.5

The discounted price = 450 – 67.5 = $382.5

20% additional discount amount on lowest price =
382.5•20/100 = $76.5

So, the final discounted price = 382.5 - 76.5 = $306.00

17. D
Original price = x,
80/100 = 12590/X,
80X = 1259000,
X = 15737.50.

18. C
Total hay = 214 kg,
The goat eats at a rate of 214/60 days = 3.6 kg per day.
The Cow eats at a rate of 214/15 = 14.3 kg per day,
Together they eat 3.6 + 14.3 = 17.9 per day.
At a rate of 17.9 kg per day, they will consume 214 kg in
214/17.9 = 11.96 or 12 days approx.

19. A
25% = 25/100 = 1/4

20. C
125/100 = 1.25

21. D
40/100 = 30/X = 40X = 30 * 100 = 3000/40 = 75

22. B
12.5/100 = 50/X = 12.5X = 50 * 100 = 5000/12.5 = 400

23. C
24/56 = 3/7 (divide numerator and denominator by 8)

24. C
Converting percent to decimal – divide percent by 100 and

remove the % sign. 87% = 87 / 100 = .87

25. A
60 has the same relation to X as 75 to 100 – so
60/X = 75/100
6000 = 75X
X = 80

26. D
60 has the same relationship to 100 as 12 does to X – so
60/100 = 12/X
1200 = 60X
X = 20

27. C
Converting a fraction into a decimal – divide the numerator by the denominator – so 71/1000 = .071. Dividing by 1000 moves the decimal point 3 places.

28. C
4.7 + .9 + .01 = 5.61

29. A
.33 × .59 = .1947

30. D
.84 ÷ .7 = 1.2

31. C
9 is in the ten thousandths place in 1.7389.

32. A
.87 - .48 = .39

33. A
Step 1: Set up the formula to calculate the dose to be given in mg as per weight of the child:-
Dose ordered X Weight in Kg = Dose to be given
Step 2: 100 mg X 23 kg = 2300 mg
(Convert 50 lb to Kg, 1 lb = 0.4536 kg, hence 50 lb = 50 X 0.4536 = 22.68 kg approx. 23 kg)
2300 mg/230 mg X 1 tablet/1 = 2300/230 = 10 tablets

34. B
1000 units/5000 units X 1 ml/1 = 1000/5000 = 0.2 ml

35. C
4 x 4 x 4 = 64

36. D
5 ml/15 ml kX 1 tsp/1 = 5/15 = 0.3 tsp

37. B
70 mg/1000 mg X 1 ml/1 = 70/1000 – 0.07 ml
(Convert 1 g = 1000 mg)
38. C
200 mg/400 mg X 1 tsp/1 = 200/400 = 0.5 tsp

39. D
600 mg/ 200 mg X 1 tablet/1 = 600/200 = 3 tablets.

40. A
At 100% efficiency 1 machine produces 1450/10 = 145 m of cloth.

At 95% efficiency, 4 machines produce 4•145•95/100 = 551 m of cloth.

At 90% efficiency, 6 machines produce 6•145•90/100 = 783 m of cloth.

Total cloth produced by all 10 machines = 551 + 783 = 1334 m

Since the information provided and the question are based on 8 hours, we did not need to use time to reach the answer.

41. C
1 foot = 12 inches, 60 feet = 60 x 12 = 720 inches.

42. A
1 centimeter = 10 millimeter, 25 centimeter = 25 X 10 = 250 millimeters.

43. A
1 millimeter = 10 centimeter, 100 millimeter = 100/10 = 10 centimeters.

44. C
1 gallon = 4 quarts, 3 gallons = 3 x 4 = 12 quarts.

45. A
There are 1000 mm in a meter, so 2000 mm = 2000/1000 = 2 meters. To divide by 1000, move the decimal 3 places to the left.

46. B
There are 1000 ml in a liter. 0.05/1000 = 0.00005 liters. To divide by 1000, move the decimal 3 places to the left.

47. D
There are 1000 mg in a gram. 30/1000 = 0.03 grams. To divide by 1000, move the decimal 3 places to the left. =

48. A
There are 10 mm in a cm. 0.101/10 = .0101. To divide by 10, move the decimal 1 place to the left.

49. B
There are 52 cards in total. Smith has 16 cards in which he can win. Therefore, his probability of winning in a single game will be 16/52. Simon has 20 winning cards so his probability of winning in single draw is 20/52.

50. B
The formula of the volume of cylinder is = $\pi r^2 h$
Where π is 3.142, r is radius of the cross sectional area, and h is the height.
So the volume will be = $3.142 \times 2.5^2 \times 12 = 235.65 m^3$.

Section III – English Grammar

1. D
The preposition "to" is correct. "To" here means give.

2. A
"Lie" means to recline, and does not take an object. "lay" means to place and does take an object.

3. A
Past unreal conditional. Takes the form,
[If ... Past Perfect ..., ... would have + past participle ...]

4. B
This sentence is in the present tense, so "to find" is correct.

5. B
The comma separates a phrase.

6. B
Words such as neither, each, many, either, every, everyone, everybody and any should take a singular pronoun.

7. D
When talking about something that didn't happen in the past, use the past perfect (if I had done).

8. C
"Lie" means to recline, and does not take an object. "Lay" means to place and does take an object. Peter lay the books on the table (the books are the direct object), or the telephone poles were lying on the road (no direct object).

9. A
Titles of short stories are enclosed in quotation marks.

10. C
No additional punctuation is required here.
11. B
Here the word "sale" is used as a "word" and not as a word in the sentence, so quotation marks are used.

12. C
Titles of short stories are enclosed in quotation marks, and commas always go inside quotation marks.

13. B
"Ran well" is correct. "Ran good" is never correct.

14. D
Commas and periods always go inside quotation marks. Question marks that are part of a quote also go inside quo-

tation marks; however, if the writer quotes a statement as part of a larger question, the question mark is placed after the quotation mark.

15. D
The sentence starts with a phrase, which is separated by a comma and then lists the things the speaker's mother taught, to say thank you, etc. Each of the items in the list are separated by a comma.

16. A
When referring to a person, use "who" instead of "that."

17. A
The comma separates a phrase starting with 'which.'

18. A
"Being honest," present tense is the best choice. "The buyer" is singular so use "is."

19. C
The subject in the first phrase, "the boy," has to agree with the subject in the second phrase, "he is."

20. D
The third conditional is used for talking about an unreal situation (a situation that did not happen) in the past. For example, "If I had studied harder, [if clause] I would have passed the exam" [main clause]. This has the same meaning as, "I failed the exam, because I didn't study hard enough."

21. B
In double negative sentences, one negative is replaced with "any."

22. B
Words such as neither, each, many, either, every, everyone, everybody and any should take a singular pronoun. Here we are assuming that the subject is male, and so use "his." The subject could be female, in which case we would use "her," however that is not one of the choices in this case.

23. B
Use "could," the past tense of "can" to express ability or capacity.

24. D
The present perfect tense cannot be used with specific time expressions such as yesterday, one year ago, last week, when I was a child, at that moment, that day, one day, etc. The present perfect tense is used with unspecific expressions such as ever, never, once, many times, several times, before, so far, already, yet, etc.

25. B
When you use 'each other' it should be used for two things or people. When you use 'one another' it should be used for things and people above two.

26. C
The verb rise ('to go up', 'to ascend.') can appear in three forms, rise, rose, and risen. The verb should not take an object.

27. B
"Went" is used in the simple past tense. "Gone" is used in the past perfect tense.

28. C
The verb raise ('to increase', 'to lift up.') can appear in three forms, raise, raised and raised.

29. C
The verb raise ('to increase', 'to lift up.') can appear in three forms, raise, raised and raised.

30. A
Words such as neither, each, many, either, every, everyone, everybody and any should take a singular pronoun.

31. D
"It's" is a contraction for it is or it has. "Its" is a possessive pronoun.

32. C
A verb can fit any of the two subjects in a compound sen-

tence while the verb form agrees with that subject.

33. A
"There" indicates a state of existence. "Their" is used for third person plural possession. "They're" is the contraction of "they are."

34. C
The two verbs "shall" and "will" should not be used in the same sentence when referring to the same future.

35. A
The verb LAY should always take an object. Here the subject is the table. The three forms of the verb lay are: lay, laid and laid. The sentence above is in past tense.

36. C
"Your" is the possessive form of "you." "You're" is the contraction of "you are."

37. A
Words such as, neither, each, many, either, every, everyone, everybody and any should take a singular pronoun.

38. B
"Lose" is a verb meaning to misplace something or to fail at a competition. "Loose" is an adjective meaning untied or able to move freely.

39. D
"Prosecute" means to begin legal proceedings against an individual or group. "Persecute" is to harass.

40. A
"Precede" means to go first or in front of others. "Proceed" means to go forward, or to begin something.

41. C
"Rise," like other intransitive verbs, is used without an object; the subject does the action on its own. For example, "The sun rises." "Raise" is a transitive verb, and is used for actions that cannot be done by a subject alone but needs an object. For example, "The student raised her hand."

42. C
The simple past tense, "had," is correct because it refers to completed action in the past.

43. C
The superlative, "hottest," is used when expressing a temperature greater than that of anything to which it is being compared.

44. B
"Cowardly" is an adjective used to modify a person.

45. A
"Deny" means to reject or disagree with the truth of something. "Refuse" means to decline to do or accept something.

46. B
"Cleverest" is the superlative form, and means the most clever.

47. B
The past perfect continuous, "has been living," is correct since the action began in the past and continues to the present.

48. B
"Please excuse my being late" has the same meaning as "Please excuse me for being late," and is correct.

49. A
Shows agreement with a negative statement by using "neither."

50. C
Doesn't, does not, or does is used with the third person singular--the pronouns he, she, and it. Don't, do not, or do is used with first, second, and third person plural.

Section IV - Vocabulary

1. B
Heinous: adj. shocking, terrible or wicked.

2. A
Harbinger: n. a person of thing that tells or announces the coming of someone or something

3. B
Judicious: Having, or characterized by, good judgment or sound thinking.

4. B
Ethanol: n. a colorless volatile flammable liquid C2H6O.

5. A
Respiratory: adj. Of, relating to, or affecting respiration or the organs of respiration.

6. B
Inherent: Naturally a part or consequence of something.

7. A
Vapid: adj. tasteless or bland.

8. C
Waif: n. homeless child or stray.

9. D
Homologous: adj. similar or identical.

10. B
Obsolete: adj. no longer in use; gone into disuse; disused or neglected.

11. A
Rankle: v. To cause irritation or deep bitterness.

12. D
Reusable

13. C
Torpid: adj. Lazy, lethargic or apathetic.

14. A
Gregarious: adj. Describing one who enjoys being in crowds and socializing.

15. B
Mutation: n. a change or alteration.

16. C
Lithe: adj. flexible or pliant.

17. A
Resent: v. to express displeasure or indignation.

18. A
Immaterial: adj. irrelevant not having substance or matter.

19. A
Impeccable: adj. perfect, no faults or errors.

20. B
Pudgy: adj. fat, plump or overweight.

21. C
Alloy: v. Mix or combine; often used of metals.

22. B
Combustible: adj. Able to catch fire and burn easily.

23. C
Salient: adj. Worthy of note; pertinent or relevant.

24. B
Ulterior: adj. beyond what is obvious or evident.

25. D
Junta: n. ruling council of a military government.

26. C
Laggard: n. someone who takes more time than necessary.

27. B
Languid: adj. lacking enthusiasm, strength or energy.

28. D
Conclusive: adj. Providing an end to something; decisive.

29. D
Mollify: v. To ease a burden; make less painful; to comfort.

30. C
Redundant: adj. Unnecessary repetition.

31. D
Raucous: adj. harsh or rough sounding.

32. D
Magnate: n. a person of influence, rank or distinction.

33. B
Liquidate: v. to convert assets into cash.

34. A
Hoax: n. To deceive (someone) by making them believe something which has been maliciously or mischievously fabricated.

35. C
Bicker: n. To quarrel in a tiresome, insulting manner.

36. C
Malady: n. A disease or ailment.

37. B
Grovel: To abase oneself before another person.

38. A
Maverick: n. Showing independence in thoughts or actions.

39. C
Nuptial: adj. Of or pertaining to wedding and marriage.

40. A
Ostensible: adj. meant for open display; apparent.

41. B
Nonchalant: adj. Casually calm and relaxed.

42. B
Pulverize: v. to completely destroy, especially by crushing to fragments or a powder.

43. D
Tenuous: adj. Thin in substance or consistency.

44. C
Octavo: n. A sheet of paper 7 to 10 inches high and 4.5 to 6 inches wide, the size varying with the large original sheet used to create it. Made by folding the original sheet three times to produce eight leaves.

45. A
Stagnant: adj. lacking freshness, motion, flow, progress, or change; stale; motionless; still.

46. D
Rebuff: n. a sudden resistance or refusal.

47. A
Pandemonium: n. Chaos; tumultuous or lawless violence.

48. A
Perpetual: adj. Continuing uninterrupted.

49. A
Pallid: adj. Appearing weak, pale, or wan.

50. A
Reimburse: v. To compensate with pay or money; especial-

ly, to repay money spent on one's behalf.

Section V – Science

1. A
The formula for acceleration = A = $(V_f - V_o)/t$
so A = $(0 - 12)/60$ sec = -0.2 m/sec^2

2. A
The Law of Multiple Proportions states that when two elements combine with each other to form more than one compound, the weights of one element that combine with a fixed weight of the other are in a ratio of small whole numbers.

3. D
All of the above are true. Electrons play an essential role in electricity, magnetism, and thermal conductivity.

4. D
An idea concerning a phenomena and possible explanations for that phenomena is an hypothesis.

5. D
All of the above. Chromosomes are

      a. Structures in a cell nucleus that carry genetic material.
      b. Consist of thousands of DNA strands.
      c. Total 46 in a normal human cell.

6. D
All of the statements about bases are true.

      a. A compound that reacts with an acid to form a salt.

      b. A molecule or ion that captures hydrogen ions.

      c. A molecule or ion that donates an electron pair to form a chemical bond.

7. D
The circulatory system disease that is one of the most frequent causes of death in North America is heart disease.

8. B
Speed = (total distance traveled)/(total time taken)
X = 1000m/20 minutes
X = 50 meters

9. A
A chemical compound is a chemical substance comprising atoms from two or more elements in a specific ration as expressed in the chemical formula i.e., H2O

10. C
The plasma membrane or cell membrane protects the cell from outside forces. It consists of the lipid bilayer with embedded proteins

11. C
Protein biosynthesis is defines as, ribosomes synthesizing proteins in the endoplasmic reticulum. This process, also known as protein biosynthesis, is a process within the cell by which the substrates convert to products of higher complexity.

12. A
Cell fractionation. Fractionation is important because it purifies the cell and its parts.

13. A
The Strong Nuclear Force is an attractive force that binds protons and neutrons and maintains the structure of the nucleus, and the Weak Nuclear Force is responsible for the radioactive beta decay and other subatomic reactions.

Note: The Weak Nuclear Force is so named because it is only effective for short distances. Nevertheless, it is through the Weak Nuclear Force that the sun provides us with energy by allowing one element to change into another element. [18]

14. B
Force = Mass times Acceleration Measured in Newtons.
1000 = 500 x A
A = 1000/500 = 2 m/s^2

15. D
Qualitative research deals with the quality, type or components of a group, substance, or mixture.

16. B

When a measurement is recorded, it includes the significant figures, which are all the digits that are certain plus
one uncertain digit.

17. B

The equation $E = mc^2$ is based on the Law of Conservation
of Mass and Energy, and   states that Energy equals
Mass times the Velocity of light^2.

18. A

A pH indicator measures hydrogen ions in a solution and
show pH on a color scale.

19. B

Acids turns blue litmus paper red, base turns red litmus
paper blue.

20. A

Covalent bonds involve a complete sharing of electrons and
occurs most commonly between atoms that have partially
filled outer shells or energy levels.

21. C

A base is any substance that can accept a hydrogen ion
and can react with fats to form soaps.

22. A

Water boils at approximately 100 °C (212 °F) at standard
atmospheric pressure.

23. D

The dominant gene controls the expression of a trait.

24. D

Wavefunction is a mathematical function that gives the
amplitude of a wave as a function of position (and sometimes, as a function of time and/or electron spin).

Note: Wavefunctions are used in chemistry to represent
the behavior of electrons bound in atoms or molecules.

25. B

The vacuum of space is an environment where bacteria do
not commonly exit. The nature of outer space, including

intense cold and lack of oxygen, makes it difficult for even most bacteria to grow.

26. B
Plants and animals are kingdoms. There are six recognized kingdoms: Animalia, Plantae, Protista, Fungi, Bacteria, and Archaea.

27. B
The elements on the periodic table can be classified as metals, metalloids and non-metals. Most of the elements on the table can be classified as metals.

28. C
A catalyst is a chemical involved in, but not changed by, a chemical reaction by which chemical bonds are weakened and reactions accelerated.

29. C
Organisms grouped into the **Protista** Kingdom include all unicellular organisms lacking a definite cellular arrangement such as **bacteria** and **algae.**

30. C
All of these statements are true.

> A metal is a substance that conducts heat and electricity.
>
> A metal is shiny and reflects many colors of light, and can be hammered into sheets or drawn into wire.
>
> About 80% of the known chemical elements are metals.

31. C
The reaction of elements with low electronegativity(almost empty outer shells) with elements with high electronegativity (mostly full outer shells) gives rise to Ionic bonds.

32. D
AIDS (or Acquired Immune Deficiency Syndrome) is carried by a virus, not bacteria.

33. A
A collection of similar or like living entities. Class has the same meaning in biology as rank. Common classes or ranks include species, order, and phylum.

34. D
All of these statements are true.

> a. Prokaryotic cells include such organisms as E. coli and Streptococcus.

> b. Prokaryotic cells lack internal membranes and organelles.

> c. Prokaryotic cells break down food using cellular respiration and fermentation.

35. B
Force = Mass times Acceleration Measured in Newtons.
$1000 = 500 \times A$
$A = 1000/500 = 2 \text{ m/s}^2$

36. B
The process of converting observed phenomena into data is called measurement.

37. A
The Law of Multiple Proportions states that when two elements combine with each other to form more than one compound, the weights of one element that combine with a fixed weight of the other are in a ratio of small whole numbers.

38. A
Morphology is defined as the field that studies the relationship between structures in living organisms.

39. A
The mass number of an atom is the total number of particles (protons and neutrons) that make it up.

40. A
All of the statements are true.

> a. Mechanical energy is the energy that is possessed by an object due to its motion or due to its position.

> b. Mechanical energy can be either kinetic energy (energy of motion) or potential energy (stored energy of position).

> c. Objects have mechanical energy if they are in motion

41. D
In Eukaryotic cells, the cell cycle is the cycle of events involving cell division, including mitosis, cytokinesis, and interphase.

42. B
The atomic number of an element equals the number of protons in an atomic nucleus, and, along with the element symbol is one of two alternate ways to label an element.

43. A
pH is a measure of effective concentration of hydrogen ions in a solution, and is approximately related to the molarity of H+ by pH = - log [H+]

44. B
Ribonucleic acid (RNA) is a chain of nucleotides that plays an important role in the creation of new proteins.

45. C
Force = Mass times Acceleration Measured in Newtons.
F = 200 X 5 = 1000 N

46. D
The Law of Definite Proportions states that every chemical compound contains fixed and constant proportions (by weight) of its constituent elements.

47. B
Four factors that affect rates of reaction are: Temperature, particle size, concentration, and the presence of a catalyst.

48. C
Spherical bacteria are Cocci. Along with bacilli, this is one of the two major structures for bacteria.

49. A
A practical test designed with the intention that its results will be relevant to a particular theory or set of theories is an experiment.

50. B
The formula for calculating molarity when the moles of the solute and liters of the solution are given is = moles of solute/ liters of solution.
Moles of Solute = 3 moles of sugar
Solution liters = 3 liters
Molarity of solution = ?

Therefore: molarity of the solution = 3 moles of solvent/ 2 liters of solution = 1.5 M solution.

51. D

All of the statements are true.

a. Electrically charged matter is influenced by, and produces, electromagnetic fields.

b. Electric current is a movement or flow of electrically charged particles.

c. Electric potential is a fundamental interaction between the magnetic field and the presence and motion of an electric charge.

52. C

Covalent or ionic bonds are considered "strong bonds."

53. C

P = 1.5 x 18 = 27 kg x m/s into the field.

54. A

Momentum of first object = 2 x 3.5 = 7; momentum of second truck = 4.3 x 1.5 = 6.45. First truck has more momentum at 7 kg x m/s moving east.

55. D

Reliability refers to the measure of an experiment's ability to yield the same or compatible results in different clinical experiments or statistical trials.

56. A

Genes are made from a long molecule called DNA, which is copied and inherited across generations. DNA is made of simple units that line up in a particular order within this large molecule. The order of these units carries genetic information, similar to how the order of letters on a page carries information. The language used by DNA is called the genetic code, which lets organisms read the information in the genes. This information is the instructions for constructing and operating a living organism.

57. A

A higher concentration of reactants causes more effective collisions per unit time, leading to an increased reaction rate.

58. C
Each chemical element has a unique atomic number representing the number of protons in its nucleus.

59. D
All of these statements are about non-metals are true.

     a. A nonmetal is a substance that conducts heat and electricity poorly.

     b. The majority of the known chemical elements are nonmetals.

     c. A nonmetal is brittle or waxy or gaseous.

60. B
Moles of solute = ? or X
Solutions liters = 5 liters
Molarity of solution = 0.5 M

Therefore: X moles/5 liters of solution = 0.5 or X/5 = 0.5
So X = 5/0.5
X = 2.5
Mole of salt in the solution is 2.5 moles

61. A
A solution with a pH value of less than 7 is acid. A pH value of 7 is neutral.

62. D
Wavelength is defined as the distance between adjacent peaks (or adjacent troughs) on a wave.

Note: Varying the wavelength of light changes its color; varying the wavelength of sound changes its pitch.

63. D
First convert 500 g to kg = 500/1000 = 0.5 kg, momentum = 0.5 x 3.5 = 1.75 kg x m/s along the road.

64. B
A catalyst is never changed in a chemical reaction.

65. A
The prediction that an observed difference is due to chance alone and not due to a systematic cause; this hypothesis is tested by statistical analysis, and accepted or rejected is the **null hypothesis**.

66. C

In science and engineering, the **accuracy** of a measurement system is the degree of closeness of measurements of a quantity to its actual (true) value.

67. B

The horizontal rows from right to left of the periodic table are known as periods and elements on a row share the same number of electron shells.

68. D

All of the statements about solubility are correct.

a. The solubility of a substance is its concentration in a saturated solution.

b. Substances with solubilities much less than 1 g/100 mL of solvent are usually considered insoluble.

c. A saturated solution is one which does not dissolve any more solute.

69. A

A valence shell is the shell corresponding to the highest value of principal quantum number in the atom.

70. C

To calculate the Molarity of a solution when the solute is given in grams and the volume of the solution is given in milliliters, you must first **convert grams to moles, and convert volume of solution in milliliters to liters.**

71. C

Hydrogen is the first element listed on the periodic table. The atomic number for hydrogen is 1.

72. B

Vertical columns on the periodic table are called groups. There are 18 groups on the table. Elements on the same group each have the same number of electrons on their outermost shell.

73. B

The **range** of a distribution is the difference between the maximum value and the minimum value.

74. B

Formula - P= kg x m/s
= 35kg x 220 m/s
= 7700 kg x m/s east

75. C

A and B are correct.
An acid is a compound containing detachable hydrogen ions.
An acid is a compound that can accept a pair of electrons from a base.

Section VI – Anatomy and Physiology

1. A

The stomach and colon are both in the Left Upper Quadrant, together with, liver, spleen, left kidney, pancreas and large intestine.

2. B

The stomach and colon are both in the Left Upper Quadrant, together with, liver, spleen, left kidney, pancreas and large intestine.

3. A

Exercise will increase metabolism.

4. A

Nerve tissue is made up of cells known as neurons.

5. D

The dermis, which contains Collagen and Elastin, gives skin its flexibility.

6. C

It is difficult to diagnose an ailment within the musculoskeletal system because of its close proximity to other organs within the body.

7. C

Angina is frequently mistaken for a heart attack. Angina pectoris, commonly known as angina, is severe chest pain

due to ischemia (a lack of blood, thus a lack of oxygen supply) of the heart muscle, generally due to obstruction or
spasm of the coronary arteries (the heart's blood vessels).[19]

8. C
An important side-benefit of the respiratory system is the
air being expelled from the mouth allows for speaking.

9. A
The process by which the immune system adapts over time
to be more efficient in recognizing pathogens is known as
acquired immunity.

10. C
Indigestion is a common digestive affliction that most
people suffer at one time or other.

11. B
Carrying urea to the kidneys is one example of the blood
stream's part in the digestive system.

12. D
All of the above. The Large Intestine passes through all the
quadrants.

13. A
Fluid balance is important, because the human body loses
water every day through urination, perspiration, feces, and
breathing.

14. D
The human skin (integumentary) is composed of a minimum of 3 major layers of tissue, the Epidermis, the Dermis
and Hypodermis.

15. B
Acne is an example of a minor ailment of the integumentary system.

16. D
Osteoporosis is a disease of bones that leads to an increased risk of fracture. In osteoporosis the bone mineral
density (BMD) is reduced, bone micro-architecture is dete-
riorating, and the amount and variety of proteins in bone
is altered. The disease may be classified as primary type 1,

primary type 2, or secondary. [20]

17. B
High blood pressure is a more common name for the circulatory system disease known as hypertension. Hypertension (HTN) or high blood pressure is a cardiac chronic medical condition in which the systemic arterial blood pressure is elevated.

18. A
Emphysema is a long-term, progressive disease of the lungs that cause shortness of breath. In people with emphysema, the tissues necessary to support the physical shape and function of the lungs are destroyed. It is included in a group of diseases called chronic obstructive pulmonary disease or COPD (pulmonary refers to the lungs). [11]

19. B
White blood cells are an important weapon in the fight against infection.

20. D
Besides the kidney, the other major organ that takes part in the body's urinary system is the Bladder.

21. B
The bladder is a balloon shaped, muscular organ.

22. B
The appendages of the integumentary system are hair, scales, feathers, and nails.

23. B
Skin cancer is an example of a serious ailment of the integumentary system.

24. D
Cardiac dysrhythmia (also known as arrhythmia and irregular heartbeat) is a term for any of a large and heterogeneous group of conditions in which there is abnormal electrical activity in the heart. The heart beat may be too fast or too slow, and may be regular or irregular. [22]

25. B
Inflammation is an example of an early response by the immune system to infection.

Conclusion

CONGRATULATIONS! You have made it this far because you have applied yourself diligently to practicing for the exam and no doubt improved your potential score considerably! Getting into a good school is a huge step in a journey that might be challenging at times but will be many times more rewarding and fulfilling. That is why being prepared is so important.

Study then Practice and then Succeed!

Good Luck!

Register for Free Updates and More Practice Test Questions

Register your purchase at www.test-preparation.ca/register.html for fast and convenient access to updates, errata, free test tips and more practice test questions.

HESI Test Strategy

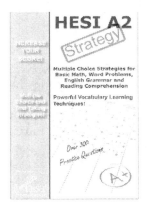

Learn and Practice Proven multiple choice strategies for Reading Comprehension, Word Problems, English Grammar and Basic Math!

If you are preparing for the Health Education Systems Exam, you probably want all the help you can get! HESI Test Strategy is your complete guide to answering multiple choice questions!

You will learn:

- Powerful multiple choice strategies with practice questions - Learn 15 powerful multiple choice strategies and then practice.

- How to prepare for a multiple choice exam

- Who does well on multiple choice exams and who does not - and how to make sure you do!

- How to handle trick questions

- Step-by-step strategy for answering multiple choice - on any subject!

- Common Mistakes on a Test - and how to avoid them

- How to avoid test anxiety

- How to prepare for a test - proper preparation for your exam will definitely boost your score!

https://www.createspace.com/4092416

Enter Code LYFZGQB5 for 25% off!

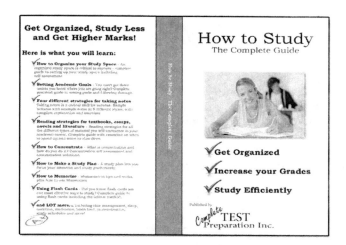

Get Organized, Study Less and Get Higher Marks!

Here is what you will learn:

- How to Organize your Study Space

- Four different strategies for taking notes

- Reading strategies for textbooks, essays, novels and literature

- How to Concentrate - What is concentration and how do you do it!

- Using Flash Cards - Complete guide to using flash cards including the Leitner method.

and LOT more... Including time management, sleep, nutrition, motivation, brain food, procrastination, study schedules and more!

Go to https://www.createspace.com/4060298

Enter Code LYFZGQB5 for 25% off!

Endnotes

Text where noted below is used under the Creative Commons Attribution-ShareAlike 3.0 License

http://en.wikipedia.org/wiki/Wikipedia:Text_of_Creative_Commons_Attribution-ShareAlike_3.0_Unported_License

1 Infectious Disease. In *Wikipedia*. Retrieved November 12, 2010 from en.wikipedia.org/wiki/Infectious_disease.

2 Virus. In *Wikipedia*. Retrieved November 12, 2010 from en.wikipedia.org/wiki/Virus.

3 Convection. In *Wikipedia*. Retrieved November 12, 2010 from en.wikipedia.org/wiki/Convection.

4 Meteorology. In *Wikipedia*. Retrieved November 12, 2010 from en.wikipedia.org/wiki/Outline_of_meteorology.

5 U.S. Navy Seal. In *Wikipedia*. Retrieved November 12, 2010 from en.wikipedia.org/wiki/United_States_Navy_SEALs.

6 Gardening. In *Wikipedia*. Retrieved January 2, 2012 from en.wikipedia.org/wiki/Gardening.

7 What Causes DNA Mutations? (n.d.) Learn.Genetics. http://learn.genetics.utah.edu/archive/sloozeworm/mutationbg.html.

8 Cell Membrane. In Wikipedia. Retrieved November 12, 2010 from http://en.wikipedia.org/wiki/Cell_membrane.

9 Spleen. In *Wikipedia*. Retrieved November 12, 2010 from http://en.wikipedia.org/wiki/Spleen.

10 Cartilage. In *Wikipedia*. Retrieved November 12, 2010 from en.wikipedia.org/wiki/Cartilage.

11 Central Nervous System. In *Wikipedia*. Retrieved November 12, 2010 from http://en.wikipedia.org/wiki/Central_nervous_system

12 Respiratory System. In *Wikipedia*. Retrieved November 12, 2010 from en.wikipedia.org/wiki/Respiratory_system.

13 Mythology. In *Wikipedia*. Retrieved November 12, 2010 from en.wikipedia.org/wiki/Mythology.

14 Insect. In *Wikipedia.* Retrieved November 12, 2010 from en.wikipedia.org/wiki/Insect.

15 Tree. In *Wikipedia.* Retrieved November 12, 2010 from en.wikipedia.org/wiki/Tree.

16 Circulatory System. In Wikipedia. Retrieved November 12, 2010 from http://en.wikipedia.org/wiki/Circulatory_system.

17 Skeletal System. In *Wikipedia.* Retrieved November 12, 2010 from http://en.wikipedia.org/wiki/Skeletal_system.

18 Nuclear Force. In *Wikipedia.* Retrieved November 12, 2010 from http://en.wikipedia.org/wiki/Nuclear_force.

19 Angina. In *Wikipedia.* Retrieved November 12, 2010 from http://en.wikipedia.org/wiki/Angina.

20 Osteoporosis. In *Wikipedia.* Retrieved November 12, 2010 from http://en.wikipedia.org/wiki/Osteoporosis.

21 Emphysema. In *Wikipedia.* Retrieved November 12, 2010 from http://en.wikipedia.org/wiki/Emphysema.

22 Cardiac Dysrhythmia. In *Wikipedia.* Retrieved November 12, 2010 from http://en.wikipedia.org/wiki/Cardiac_dysrhythmia.

CPSIA information can be obtained at www.ICGtesting.com
Printed in the USA
LVOW10s0905030416

481969LV00019B/649/P

9 781928 077572